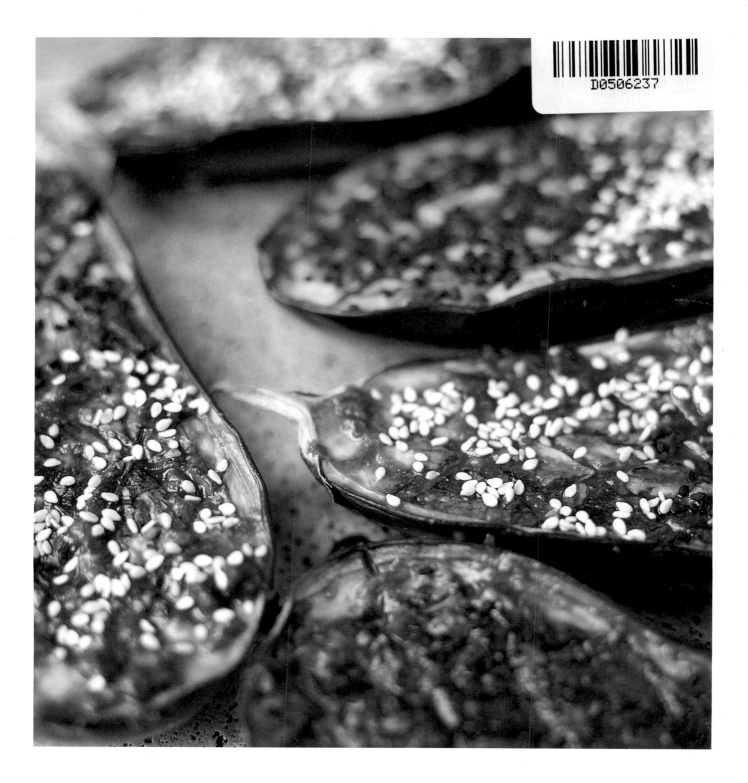

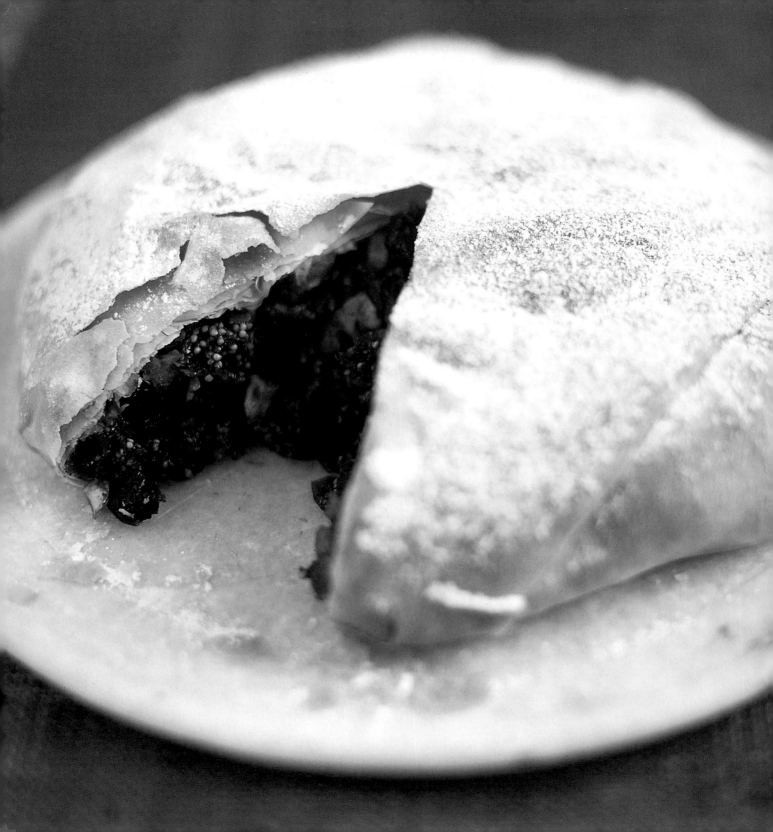

Sophie Braimbridge   Erica Jankovich RD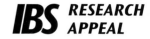

Healthy Cooking for IBS

photography by Tara Fisher

Stewart, Tabori & Chang
New York

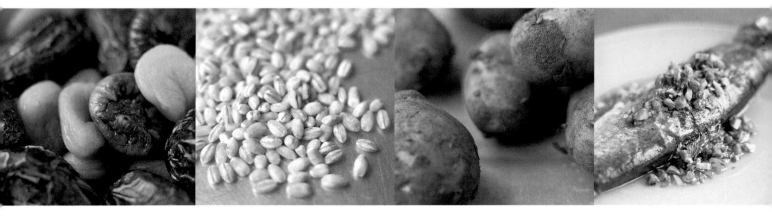

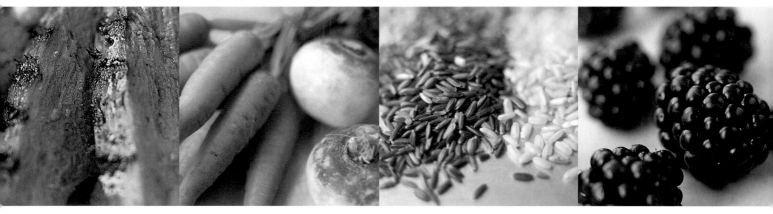

To Ab who has had to endure many a recipe test. (Sophie Braimbridge)

To my home team Jonty, Tim, and Alex for their tireless enthusiasm, encouragement and time. (Erica Jankovich)

Acknowledgments

Sophie Braimbridge:

To Muna and Jenny who have always laughed at my jokes. Thank you.

Erica Jankovich:

To Professor Silk, Wendy, and Jane for their continued support.

To John Peters and the IBS Research Appeal for believing in and promoting diet and good nutrition as a valuable part of the management of IBS.

To all my patients past and present who have given me such valuable experience.

To Sophie Braimbridge whom I thoroughly enjoyed working with and who was able to shed some wonderful insight into fiber modified dishes.

To Muna Reyal and Jenny Wheatley from Kyle Cathie for putting all this together so efficiently and producing a lifestyle cookbook that will help IBS sufferers conquer their symptoms and enjoy their food.

At any time of the day or night, one in five of us will be suffering from one or more of the many symptoms of Irritable Bowel Syndrome. IBS as it is generally known is not life threatening—but for many, it's a living nightmare with pain, bloating, urgency, diarrhea, constipation, and the embarrassment of gas and soiling being a few of the symptoms that significantly reduce the quality of life of its victims.

From a clinician's point of view, a major headache is that you can't point to a specific spot on a patient's body and say "There! That's the cause of your IBS." IBS is a "functional" disorder…its symptoms simply occur…there are no abnormalities in digestion or in the absorption of fluids and nutrients and no structural abnormalities that can be identified in the gastrointestinal tract. It comes, it goes, or it stays—sometimes for years.

Since we launched our research program through the IBS Research Appeal in 1992 we've identified stress as one of the major triggers of IBS attacks. But there's not a great deal of commonality between IBS cases—episodes can be triggered by a combination of causes, including mental, physical, and sexual abuse. They can be hormonal and cyclical…and it's equally true that in many, many instances, IBS attacks are directly related to what we eat and drink.

Because the causes are so varied, modern management strategies favor a multidisciplinary approach to treatment. These include pharmacological treatments directed toward the intestines—often combined with centrally targeted treatments to overcome psychosocial factors that play an important role in triggering attacks: treatments could include physiological explanation of symptoms, psychotherapy, hypnotherapy, cognitive behavioral therapy (C.P.T.) and for stress, the use of mild antidepressants. However, an extremely important component of the multidisciplinary approach to the management of IBS is the different dietary measures that can be applied.

This collaboration between chef Sophie Braimbridge and dietitian Erica Jankovich has produced a clear and authoritative text and wonderful recipes that I am confident will contribute greatly to the dietary management of IBS. In my experience there is no one better qualified to contribute to the field of dietary management of IBS than Erica Jankovich. For a number of years, Erica has carried out a very important role in our IBS research program and as a member of our clinical team she, more than any anyone else, understands the value of promoting relevant and healthy eating in IBS.

I also feel that this book reflects the goals of the IBS Research Appeal…we seek simply to improve the management of this very common condition. We continue to strive to understand more of the factors responsible for causing the symptoms. We continue to collaborate closely with the pharmaceutical industry in their development of new treatments for IBS and we continue to research and promote dietary measures that can help IBS sufferers. The IBS Research Appeal has always assumed educational responsibilities toward IBS sufferers and during our studies, we have published bulletins, newsletters and books about the condition. These, along with our book *Understanding Your Irritable Bowel,* generate income that allows us to continue our research. Our latest innovation is our website: www.please-help-my-ibs.org, which we invite you to visit. It offers a question and answer facility that is providing us with more information about the condition while enabling us to address specific questions from sufferers. The IBS Research Appeal is pleased to be associated with this valuable and helpful book.

Professor David Silk MD, FRCP, Director of Research, IBS Research Appeal

Introduction

If you suffer from Irritable Bowel Syndrome (IBS), you will be pleased to know that you are not alone. Although it is difficult to talk about, if you did broach the subject with your family, friends, and colleagues, you would discover that IBS affects us all at some stage in our life to a lesser or greater degree.

We are not machines; no one's bowels are always regular as clockwork. We all have experienced excessive gas, bloating, abdominal pain, urgency, constipation, and diarrhea at some stage in the past year.

Statistics vary from source to source, but it does seem clear that IBS is more prevalent in the modern world than in developing countries. At any one time IBS has been said to affect up to 25 percent of people living in the West. We know that of diagnosed sufferers 60–65 percent are female and 35–40 percent are male. It is also more prevalent in young adults and most commonly associated with life-changing, stressful events.

To a large extent IBS is a hidden disease, classified in the medical world as a functional gastrointestinal disorder, meaning that it is not caused by a specific organic disease but rather by a combination of certain symptoms. Many sufferers tend to go undiagnosed for a long time before they go to a doctor. When they do reach the doctor, it is still difficult for the average general practitioner to put the puzzle together. Some patients have reported that it has taken three visits to different practitioners before the diagnosis was

made. There are reports of people who have suffered for five to ten years before seeking help.

The impact of IBS can vary from person to person and from day to day and month to month. Symptoms can range from mildly inconvenient to severely debilitating. IBS can frustrate your emotional, social, and professional life. It may result in absences from work and social functions and can also limit your ability to take part in sports and leisure activities.

The good news is that help is available. Although IBS is a recognized and complex condition, we know that it is treatable. Because of this complexity, it is important not to self-diagnose, and although you may think many of your symptoms match those you read about in this and indeed other books, it is important that you visit a properly qualified and experienced doctor.

Your first port of call is your local doctor, who may refer you to a gastrointestinal specialist. You will receive a full medical run-down, resulting in a clear individual diagnosis. The specialist will then begin treatment, which could involve medication and referral to a specialist dietitian and/or psychologist. Because of its nature and complexity, treatments for IBS can be rather varied. One American survey conducted by the International Foundation for Functional Gastrointestinal Disorders published in 2004 cited the use of 281 different treatments, including drugs, over-the-

counter medications, and herbal and dietary supplements. Not nearly as extreme, this section of this book will examine:

- ▶ The disease, including symptoms and a susceptibility test for you to complete.
- ▶ The respective treatments and a holistic approach to treating IBS.
- ▶ General dietary principles and the application of diet to managing and controlling IBS.
- ▶ The alternative approaches to treating IBS.

Essentially, this book acts as both a dietary manual and cookbook, guiding you through the different stages of the dietary treatment for your particular type of IBS. Each of the recipes has been specifically developed and scientifically analyzed to enable you to build them into your specific IBS diet. However, as explained later on, managing and controlling IBS should be holistic, drawing on a combination of professional medical guidance, lifestyle improvement, and specific dietary management.

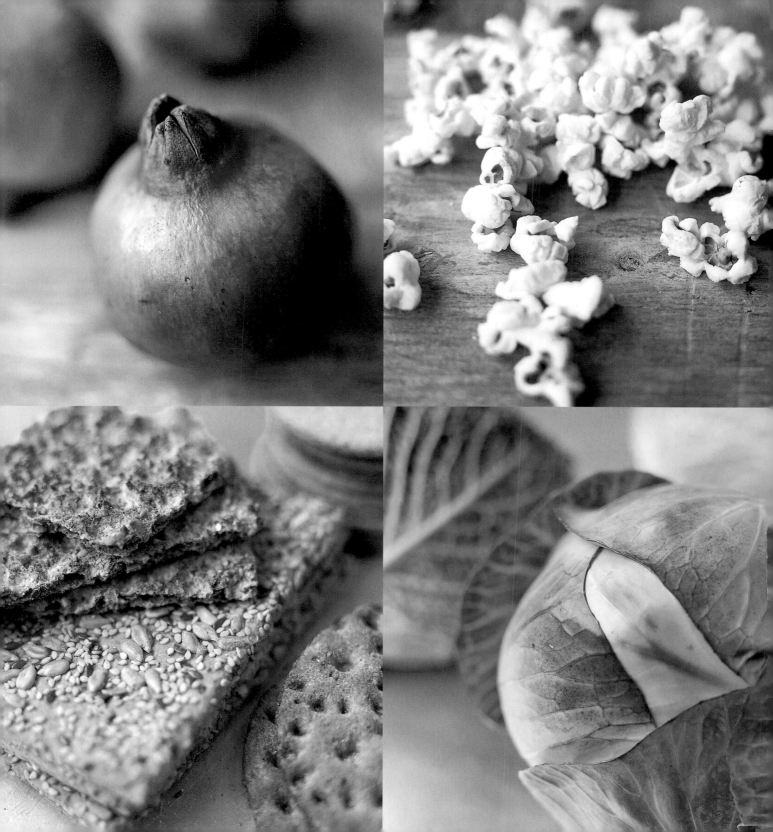

About IBS

The digestive system

Food and drink move progressively from the mouth down through the esophagus (gullet) into the stomach, where they are held for a while to allow a certain amount of digestion to take place. They then move into the intestines where they mix with other digestive juices, slowly but consistently passing through the small and then the large bowel. Most nutrient absorption takes place in the small intestine. Nutrients then move from here through the gut wall into the bloodstream where they are transported around the body to be utilized or broken down for excretion. Fluid is slowly reabsorbed in the large bowel, particularly the colon, allowing the stool to form and subsequently be passed. This natural process of the movement of food through the digestive tract is made possible by contraction and relaxation of the muscles lining it, a process known as peristalsis or gut motility.

So what goes wrong in the digestive system of the IBS sufferer? Latest research into IBS seems to indicate that symptoms usually arise from a combination of the following:

▶ Certain microscopic structural abnormalities in the gut lining. It is not yet clear what leads to these abnormalities.
▶ The influence of psychological factors, resulting in heightened sensitivity to pain and changes in normal bowel movement.

Symptoms and signs

Examination by a qualified medical practitioner is important as many symptoms of IBS can mirror those of other bowel diseases. The doctor, if they feel it necessary, will carry out blood tests, an endoscopy (a procedure where a tiny camera is inserted into your digestive tract and the lining of your bowel wall can be examined), x-rays and other tests to rule out other bowel diseases. In the IBS patient no obvious abnormality will be revealed, and this in itself is often a relief for the sufferer. IBS is therefore classified as a functional disorder of the bowel, meaning that it relates to disturbance of the bowel's normal functioning without resulting from any change in the bowel's structure or from any obvious cause.

The symptoms of IBS can be physical or neurological in nature.

Physical symptoms

Further explanation of each of the more common physical symptoms is set out below.

Crampy abdominal pain

It is evident that most IBS sufferers experience this symptom. The region of the bowel affected by pain can vary from person to person. When the bowel attempts to move its contents through, the process called peristalsis (described above) is started by contraction of the muscles lining the abdominal wall.

In the IBS sufferer's bowel there seems to be abnormal movement or

Physical symptoms include:
▶ Crampy abdominal pain
▶ Change in bowel habit; constipation, diarrhea, alternating between the two
▶ Mucus
▶ Gas, flatulence, and bloating
▶ Urgency, incontinence
▶ Incomplete bowel movement
▶ Belching
▶ Nausea
▶ Indigestion

Neurological symptoms include:
▶ Anxiety
▶ Depression
▶ Headaches and dizziness
▶ Joint pain
▶ Muscle fatigue
▶ Lack of energy

contraction of the bowel wall as it attempts to move the contents through, and this is what causes the pain. It is also clear from available research that IBS patients have a more sensitive gut with a lower pain threshold than in unaffected people, and this is another reason for their experiencing more marked pain.

Change in bowel habit

Constipation

Constipation means the passage of small, hard and infrequent stools. Some IBS sufferers pass small stools daily, others open their bowels once a week. The condition is often associated with pain and abdominal discomfort, and many sufferers also experience the feeling of incomplete evacuation.

Constipation can occur for a number of reasons. A proper medical examination is necessary to ascertain whether the problem is purely diet-related, or whether it is due to a mechanical obstruction or muscular defect.

Diarrhea

This means the passage of rapid, loose, watery stools through the colon. In the IBS patient this is likely to be due to an abnormal increase in motility of fluid content (meaning the body is producing more fluid via movement from the tissues into the gut). Diarrhea is a significant change in normal bowel function, so make sure you can describe your symptoms in detail to your doctor as this can also be an indicator of other gastrointestinal diseases.

Alternating bowel habit

Some IBS sufferers experience what we call alternating bowel habit, meaning that they will go through a period of constipation and then suddenly get a rush of diarrhea for a few days and then find themselves constipated again.

Mucus

This is produced in the lining of the colon. It acts as a lubricant and a transport medium for the enzymes necessary for digestion. In some IBS patients, due to the increase in contractility, more mucus is produced and can be seen in the stool.

Gas, flatulence, and bloating

The gases in our bowel come from what we swallow and the changes that occur to certain foods when they are eaten. Healthy gut bacteria metabolize a type of fiber called soluble fiber (found mainly in fruit and vegetables) to produce energy that can be used by the body and gases. Gases are in most cases hydrogen, carbon dioxide, and methane. It has been proved that in certain IBS patients who harbor excessive amounts of sulphur-producing bacteria, extra gases such as hydrogen sulphide and methanethiol are also produced, which result in the passage of foul-smelling flatus (bad smelly gas). The short-chain fatty acids act as a fuel source, thus feeding the colonic bacteria to increase their quantity and fermentation rate and therefore to increase production of these bowel gases. So the more bacteria you feed with soluble fiber, the more gases are produced.

The disturbed gut motility patterns that are commonly seen in IBS patients result in poor movement of these gases as well as of solid matter through the bowel. Research has indeed shown that gases tend to move both up and down the bowel, and they have also been seen to accumulate in sections which could give rise to bloating and pain. In some IBS patients, bloating and gas are caused by the inability to move gas properly through the bowel.

Most IBS patients experience bloating and report that it occurs mainly after a meal and progressively worsens as the day moves on. Many also say that it settles after a night's sleep.

Urgency, incontinence

You may also find yourself dashing to the bathroom with little and unsatisfactory results. Urgency is common in IBS and mainly due to a hypersensitivity of the muscles of the rectum. Some people with IBS will also suffer the embarrassment of soiling.

Incomplete bowel movement

This refers to the feeling that when you have opened your bowels you are not yet finished.

Belching

In some IBS patients excessive burping is common. The anxious IBS patient tends to be more susceptible. Usually belching is a natural process and does not indicate that there is a problem with digestion; however it can become excessive and can be worsened by stress. There are some schools of thought that believe it is a learned reaction to the ingestion of food. Measures such as eating slowly, avoiding carbonated drinks, caffeine, and chewing gum are sometimes recommended. Stress reduction and relaxation seem to be of more benefit.

Nausea

The urge to vomit is often experienced by IBS patients. It is said to be due to a slow rate of stomach emptying, particularly in post-infective IBS patients (see page 13), but has also been attributed to enhanced gut sensitivity, which is common in all sufferers.

Indigestion

Dyspepsia or indigestion is brought about by the ultra-sensitive lining of the IBS patient's bowel. Food is ingested as normal, but because of their enhanced gut sensitivity levels, IBS sufferers will experience fullness, sensitivity, and indigestion much sooner than non-sufferers.

Neurological symptoms

Some patients experience severely debilitating symptoms not related to their gut. These include problems with an irritable bladder and passing urine, and gynecological symptoms specifically associated with the female menstrual cycle.

Anxiety and depression

IBS sufferers are often worriers—they have the type of personality which is easily affected by stress. The development of IBS or the worsening of symptoms is often associated with a stressful event or a change in life circumstances.

Research has shown that IBS patients are generally more concerned and obsessed than average about their body functions and the possibility of illness and disease. Disturbances in mood, such as depression and anxiety, can influence the functioning of the bowel. Chemical changes that occur in the brain can affect the gut via a pathway known as the brain-gut axis, resulting in heightened sensitivity to pain and changes in normal bowel movement.

Headaches and dizziness, joint pain, muscle fatigue, and lack of energy

These are all well recognized as symptoms of IBS but also of a disease known as fibromyalgia, which is characterized by unexplained aches, pains, and fatigue combined with neurological symptoms. A fair percentage of IBS patients may also suffer from this disease.

Fatigue and general malaise are commonly cited by IBS patients, mainly females. It seems that IBS may be related to chronic fatigue syndrome. The cause of these symptoms is not yet fully understood, although subject to much ongoing research.

What are the causes of IBS?

Many people ask how they can go through a good part of their life having absolutely no bowel complaints at all and then suddenly start developing IBS-type symptoms. There is no simple answer to this question and indeed IBS has been seen to develop for a number of reasons. It is a chronic condition, but many of its symptoms are controllable by the correct combination of diet, medication, exercise, and lifestyle management.

Poor diet

We all lead busy lives and hardly stop to put any thought into what, where, or when we are eating and drinking. The day often passes by without a sensible thought given to food. Our diet is generally low in nutrient balance and low in a suitable mix of fibers. The food we eat is often highly processed or in a reheatable or ready-made form and contains many additives. We certainly don't drink enough water. All of these factors are counterproductive to a normal, healthy, happy bowel habit.

Food intolerance

In certain instances, eating will trigger IBS symptoms. Sufferers immediately start searching for a suspected food allergy or intolerance, but blood antibody and skin-prick allergy testing have repeatedly revealed negative results. It is believed that it is not a specific food that triggers the reaction but rather a hypersensitive gut, overreacting to its contents. These noted intolerances also tend to affect IBS patients one day yet disappear the next. Studies indicate that emotional or psychological stress and tension can make the bowel more sensitive, causing it to be inconsistent in its reaction to certain foods at any given time.

Psychological factors

As mentioned above, the term brain-gut axis refers to the nerve linkages between the gut and the brain. A whole body of evidence exists to support the theory that psychological factors such as anxiety, depression, mood changes, and stress affect bowel symptoms and function. Many IBS sufferers will have experienced an episode of abdominal pain and diarrhea before a stressful event such as an exam or important game. Others will remember becoming constipated when depressed.

Poor motility

IBS patients have developed an abnormal bowel contractility cycle. Researchers believe that this is due to a microscopic structural abnormality in the lining of the gut wall where a specialized chemical involved in gut contractility is released at an abnormal rate, resulting in increased or decreased motility.

Inflammation and increased sensitivity of the gut lining

A hypersensitive gut could arise from a previous gut infection or from a stressful life event in the sufferer's past. Any food that is eaten could cause crampy abdominal pain which arises from an increased sensitivity to distension of the colon or intestines by gases and fluid.

Previous gastrointestinal infection

A previous serious gastrointestinal infection, such as salmonella or shigella, often contracted on a trip to a foreign country, has been shown to correlate closely with patients subsequently developing IBS. This is referred to as post-infective IBS. It seems that such a severe infection results in a long-term mild inflammation of the gut. The worse the infection, the higher the susceptibility of the person to developing IBS. The anxiety associated with the time of the illness probably further sensitizes the gut.

Who is susceptible?

The factors listed below have been seen to be common linkages among those developing IBS.

If you answer YES to the majority of the questions below, you are likely to be susceptible to IBS.

▶ Does anyone in your family suffer from IBS?
▶ Do any of your family suffer from constipation?
▶ Is there any history of psychiatric illness?
▶ Have you had a previous gastrointestinal infection or a serious bout of food poisoning, perhaps while traveling in another country?
▶ Have you had any previous gastrointestinal surgery?
▶ Are you female?
▶ Do you work long hours and at weekends?
▶ Is your job stressful?
▶ Is your private life stressful?
▶ Do you skip meals?
▶ Do you eat at your desk or in front of the TV?
▶ Do you drink more than three cups of caffeinated drinks per day?

If you answer NO to the majority of the questions below, it indicates further susceptibility to IBS.

▶ Do you find time to relax every day?
▶ Do you exercise regularly?
▶ Do you eat at the same time every day?
▶ Do you eat the same amount of food at every meal?
▶ Do you eat a healthy balanced diet?
▶ Does your diet contain fiber?
▶ Do you drink enough water? (See pages 32–33)

Different types of IBS

IBS as a disease has a great variety of symptoms, and treatment is made easier if we classify patients into three predominant types. Over the past 20 years there has been much debate in the medical field as to how to split these patients into different groups, but there seems now to be worldwide consensus that a symptom-based approach to diagnosis is best.

IBS is almost always associated with the crampy abdominal pain normally relieved on defecation. Patients also tend to have the feeling of incomplete bowel movement, they might pass mucus with a stool and also experience abdominal fullness, gas, bloating, or swelling. As such, patients are then categorized into those that are:

▶ Constipation predominant
▶ Diarrhea predominant
▶ Alternating type (between the above two)

Before a medical specialist can classify you, the above symptoms need to have been noticed for 12 weeks or more (which need not be consecutive) during the past year.

How is IBS Treated?

Holistic treatment

IBS is a chronic, intermittent, and relapsing functional disease. Functional gastrointestinal diseases are a group of diseases where there is no specific known identifiable cause but patients have a recognizable set of symptoms. Symptoms can overlap with those of other illnesses, so ensure that you get a proper diagnosis.

In all my experience, I have come to realize that the best approach is a multidisciplinary one. Those IBS sufferers who have examined the whole picture and devoted time to looking into and taking on board all angles of IBS treatment are those who are most successful in managing their symptoms and controlling their IBS.

The four main areas that need to be managed are your:
▶ Drug regime
▶ Lifestyle
▶ Diet
▶ Fluid intake (see pages 32–33)

It is important for the doctor and dietitian to work together as treatment by pharmacological means must occur in conjunction with dietary management. In many cases the drug treatment prescribed by your doctor will act as an interim measure while the other aspects of treatment are coming up to speed. Drug treatment tends to be either end-organ-targeted (aimed at the gut) or centrally targeted (aimed at the brain). Lifestyle management involves getting your "house" in order—having a look at how you run your life or allow your life to be run by others. It involves critically appraising your work versus your social life and leisure time. Importantly this process should also involve taking stock of your exercise and relaxation patterns.

Dietary management is very much centered around the type of IBS you have. It is based on investigating and treating the symptoms you as an individual have. It is often necessary to start by going back to basic guidelines for healthy eating. These are principles we have all learned before but as a consequence of modern living have let fall by the wayside.

Improving your fluid intake is the easiest aspect of the treatment to understand but the hardest actually to put into practice. The importance of fluid is discussed in more detail later on.

The drugs

It is important to understand that because of the variation in the way IBS affects different people, drug treatments will also affect people in different ways. Some drugs may work for you but not for your friend who also has IBS. For this reason it is important that you establish a good relationship with your treating doctor and are able to talk openly and clearly about how you feel. Also be prepared to do a little chopping and changing with drugs until you find what suits you best.

Many of the drugs used in the treatment of IBS also require that you take them consistently in order to get the desired effect, so you would need to commit to at least two or three weeks before making any decision regarding their effectiveness.

Here is a basic breakdown of the types of drugs you may be prescribed:

End-organ-targeted

▶ Anti-diarrheals—will reduce urgency, make stool output more predictable and improve consistency.
▶ Anti-spasmodics—will relax the smooth muscles in the gut, improving and moderating contractility, thereby reducing pain.
▶ Laxatives—soften the stool, making it easier to pass. They can be the bulking type, which are mainly fiber derivatives and work by retaining fluid; or they can be the osmotic type, which soften and lubricate by drawing water into the gut from the body tissues.
▶ Receptor active treatment—a revolutionary new treatment for IBS, involving a range of drugs that work on certain receptor cells lining the bowel wall by either increasing or decreasing intestinal motility and contractility.

Centrally targeted

Mild antidepressants are often used in treating IBS, especially when the brain-gut axis is very involved in its cause. Certain antidepressants are better suited to certain types of IBS, affecting the rate of movement of contents around the gut. This type of treatment should not be dismissed as an improvement in mood; stress levels and anxiety can have an important effect on bowel function and other IBS symptoms.

It is important to note, however, that drugs by themselves are not the answer. You should follow the dietary management guidelines regardless of your drug regime.

Lifestyle

Your life should take just as important a role in your treatment as does your diet and your drug regime. We all spend too much time on the go and too little time looking after ourselves. IBS is all about you and the way you do things. Have a long hard look at your lifestyle. Take active measures to change the way you live and what you do in a day. Make realistic changes that you can sustain.

Your work

How much time do you spend at work? Are you working realistic hours? Do you allow yourself a break at lunchtime or do you eat at your desk? Are you under pressure at work? On a scale of 1 to 10, how much stress are you under? All this can be changed in order to improve your health. After all, you are far more beneficial to your employer or your business when you are healthy. Think of cutting back, working from home and getting home in time for dinner with your family.

Your exercise

For some people exercise is routine, for others it is sporadic, and for others it is nonexistent. We all know that we should be exercising more, so why aren't we doing it? We need to get our priorities straight. The benefits of exercise are many, particularly in the management of IBS. Regular appropriate exercise will reduce our stress levels, improve our psychological outlook and aid the movement of stool throughout the digestive system. We need to commit time to activity: it is best achieved if it is part of our daily routine. Recent research claims that a minimum of 20 and a maximum of 60 minutes of moderate exercise a day is more beneficial than two or three visits to the gym in a week. Moderate exercise means a good, fast, purposeful walk which raises the heart rate but doesn't leave you panting. This can easily be achieved by walking to and from work or putting your sneakers on and hitting the park at lunchtime or cycling to school.

Stress, relaxation, and counseling

Just taking the first steps to investigate your problem, talking to your doctor and allowing him or her to explain the physiological basis of your symptoms will reduce your anxiety level and make you feel better. Your doctor may refer you to a psychologist for counseling, which may involve hypnotherapy, relaxation therapy, or cognitive behavioral therapy, all of which have been shown to have beneficial effects on IBS.

Allow yourself time to relax, plan it into a day. Perhaps take up a hobby or enroll yourself in a part-time course. Stop rushing: get up earlier and give yourself time at home and in the bathroom.

Diet

The way in which your diet can be managed to help your IBS depends on your individual symptoms. Research in the field is varied and in some cases inconclusive, but we do know that one diet is not suitable for all IBS sufferers. This book will help to guide you toward individualizing your dietary treatment; however, if you are not getting the expected results, please seek further guidance from a properly qualified and preferably specialized dietitian who has had experience in the area.

The available research has investigated three main areas of specific dietary management:
- Manipulation of the fiber content
- Supplementation of the diet with digestive bran
- The identification of food intolerances

Researchers are not yet agreed on the most appropriate dietary management of IBS. However, experience suggests that the best results are achieved with careful attention to the individual's symptoms and by basing the dietary treatment on improving these specific uncomfortable symptoms.

Managing Your Diet

This section of the book starts by showing you how to assess your current diet and explaining the principles of healthy and balanced eating by concentrating on "getting the basics right." It then provides insight into the manipulation and management of the fiber content of your diet according to your symptoms.

Assessing your present diet

It is essential that you take an in-depth look at your present diet before coming to any conclusions regarding how to change it to influence your IBS symptoms. Do this by keeping a careful food diary for four to seven days. Record everything that you eat and drink. In addition, record the quantities you consume as well as your associated symptoms each day. The table below represents an example of a food diary

and some guidelines as to how to complete it.

The purpose of the food diary is to estimate your dietary intake and/or to determine if you have associated symptoms with certain foods. The accuracy of the result is very much dependent on the completeness of your record, so the more days you can cover, the more accurate the result will be. It is important to:

- ▶ Try to complete a minimum of four days that are representative of your usual diet.
- ▶ Record your intake immediately after meals if possible, when it is still fresh in your mind.
- ▶ Describe all items in detail: for example, "lean shoulder of beef," not just "beef"; "skimmed milk" instead of just "milk."

- ▶ Write down brand names wherever possible.
- ▶ List quantities in detail, or use common household measures such as slices, scoops, tablespoons, and so on.
- ▶ Indicate your method of cooking: for instance battered cod, boiled rice.
- ▶ List the ingredients if a dish contains more than one ingredient.
- ▶ Keep the labels from all preprepared meals you eat.
- ▶ Record how much fat and oil you use when cooking.

Once you have completed the diary you need to make a summary of it and consider whether your eating habits are meeting basic healthy-eating guidelines. Do this by referring to the dietary assessment table opposite to compare your present dietary intake to your recommended intake.

Example of a food diary

DAY	TIME	FOOD ITEM	DESCRIPTION	AMOUNT	FLUID	SYMPTOMS
Monday	8 a.m.	Orange juice	Fresh (carton)		³/₄ cup	Indigestion
		Tea	With milk		2 cups	
		Milk	Full-fat	²/₃ cup	In cereal	
		Sugar		2 teaspoons		
		Cereal	Bran flakes	5 tablespoons		
		Toast	Wholewheat bread	1 slice		
		Margarine	Polyunsaturated light	Medium amount spread		
		Jelly	Strawberry	1 teaspoon		

Dietary assessment table

QUESTION	ANSWER	RECOMMENDED PER DAY	EXPLANATION	BENEFITS
How many meals a day did you eat?		3 meals	3 meals per day should be enough for most of us. In special medical circumstances you may require smaller meals, but never skip a meal.	Regular meals help increase our metabolic rate, regulate our blood sugar, and help our bowels to function at regular intervals.
How many hours were there between each meal?		4–6 hours	Try to eat your meals at evenly spaced intervals of 4–6 hours every day. Do not eat too late or too early.	We are creatures of habit. Regular meals at evenly spaced intervals will help create a regular bowel habit. Eating too early or too late will upset this balance.
How many snacks did you eat?		0–2	It is best from a weight-control perspective if you can get by without snacking. However, if you are going to snack, make it healthy and low in fat.	Calorie intake is better controlled if you can avoid snacking.
How many portions of fruit and vegetables did you eat?		4–5	Eat 5 in total per day. Fruit juice and beans and pulses can count only as one portion each per day.	Vitamin C, carotene, folates, calcium, and iron, fiber, and some carbohydrates, plus phytochemicals and antioxidants (cancer-protective compounds).
How many times a day did you eat carbohydrates (breads, pasta, rice, potatoes, and cereals)?		3	Starchy, high-fiber carbohydrates, such as cereals, bread, pasta, rice, and potatoes, should make up 50% of each meal.	Carbohydrates for energy, fiber, B vitamins, calcium and iron.
How big were your portions of protein (meat, fish, and chicken) at your main meal?		Meat: 3–4oz. Fish: 5oz. Chicken: 4oz. Pulses, soy: 5oz.	Stick to smaller portions of low-fat protein on which there is no obvious fat, e.g. skinless chicken or trimmed bacon.	Iron, protein, B vitamins including B^{12}, zinc, and magnesium.
How many times did you eat/drink milk, cheese, or yogurt?		2–3	Eating low-fat dairy products 2–3 times per day (glass of milk, matchbox of cheese, small yogurt) should ensure a high enough calcium intake.	Calcium, protein, vitamins B12 and B^2, vitamins A and D.
Did you eat chips, chocolate, or sweets?		0–1	Obviously, the less you eat of these, the better.	Empty calories, no real nutritional value.
How many teaspoons of margarine, butter, or oil did you use?		3–4	Choose low-fat varieties that are olive oil based for better heart health.	Essential fatty acids, fat-soluble vitamins D and E.
How many teaspoons of sugar did you use?		0	Be aware of food and drink containing sugar: they contribute to weight gain and tooth decay.	Empty calories!
What did you drink? Water Tea Coffee Alcohol (units)		Water: 3½ pints per day Tea/coffee: 3–4 cups per day Alcohol: 2–3 units for women and 3–4 units for men (on 4–5 days per week)	Keep dehydrating drinks like caffeine-based fluids and alcohol to a minimum. Always drink lots of water every day.	Hydration (see page 32).

A balanced diet

Once you have assessed how you are doing, the first step in dietary management for all IBS patients is to get basic eating patterns right. Learn to eat the right nutrients in the right proportions.

All over the world the theory of basic healthy eating is the same. Wherever you come from, the authorities on nutrition are all promoting the "five food group" theory. The five food groups are:

Carbohydrates

▶ Carbohydrate, dietary fiber, calcium, and some vitamins such as B vitamins and iron are supplied by this group.
▶ Carbohydrates can be broken down into two basic groups. Simple carbohydrates are more refined and sugary and require minimal digestion to break them down. Complex carbohydrates are unrefined or contain a larger percentage of fiber; these take longer to metabolize.
▶ All carbohydrates are broken down in the bowel to glucose to supply energy.
▶ Breads, rice, cereal, pasta, and grains fall within this group.
▶ Eat starch at every meal.
▶ Have 6–11 portions in total per day. See page 21 for recommended portion sizes.

Fruit and vegetable group

▶ Fruits and vegetables provide vitamins, minerals, carbohydrates, and fiber.

Vitamin C is necessary to build the structure of cells and tissues; it aids wound healing and iron absorption; along with carotene and vitamin A it protects against chronic diseases.
▶ Eat this group fresh, dried, canned, frozen, or in the form of juice.
▶ Have 5 servings per day. See page 21 for recommended portion sizes.

Protein group

▶ Protein-rich foods are essential for growth and repair of the body.
▶ Protein also supplies iron, B vitamins, zinc, and magnesium, which are all essential for the formation of blood products, the strengthening of the immune system, and the healing of wounds.
▶ Animal protein is found in meat, fish, and poultry.
▶ Plant protein is found in nuts, seeds, pulses, and TVP (textured vegetable protein, such as soy).
▶ Have 2–3 servings per day. See page 21 for recommended portion sizes.

Dairy group

▶ Dairy products provide calcium, protein and vitamin B^{12}, and vitamins A and D.
▶ Calcium is essential, helping to build strong teeth and bones.
▶ This group includes all milk and milk derivatives such as cheeses and yogurt.
▶ Have 2–3 servings per day. See page 21 for recommended portion sizes.

A note on plant proteins

The soybean is an excellent source of protein, being low in fat and containing no cholesterol. Soybeans have also been shown to have anticarcinogenic properties. Most importantly for IBS patients, soy and its products contain fiber. TVP (textured vegetable protein) is a soy derivative that has been processed to resemble meat.

Tofu is the curd part of coagulated soy milk sometimes known as bean curd; it can be bought as a solid block or as a soft, cream-like substance, and can be used in stir-fries, salads or casseroles or as a dip or spread.

Tempeh and miso are fermented soy bean pastes, miso having the addition of grains such as barley or rice during fermentation; they can be cooked in a variety of ways.

Fats and sugars

▶ Simple sugars are considered empty energy as they supply only glucose, with no vitamins and minerals. Fats supply energy in the form of fat as well as fat-soluble vitamins which are important for the health of our cell walls and tissues.
▶ Keep the intake of these to a minimum.
▶ To ensure good heart health, concentrate on having mainly monounsaturated fats in your diet, such as olive oil based products.

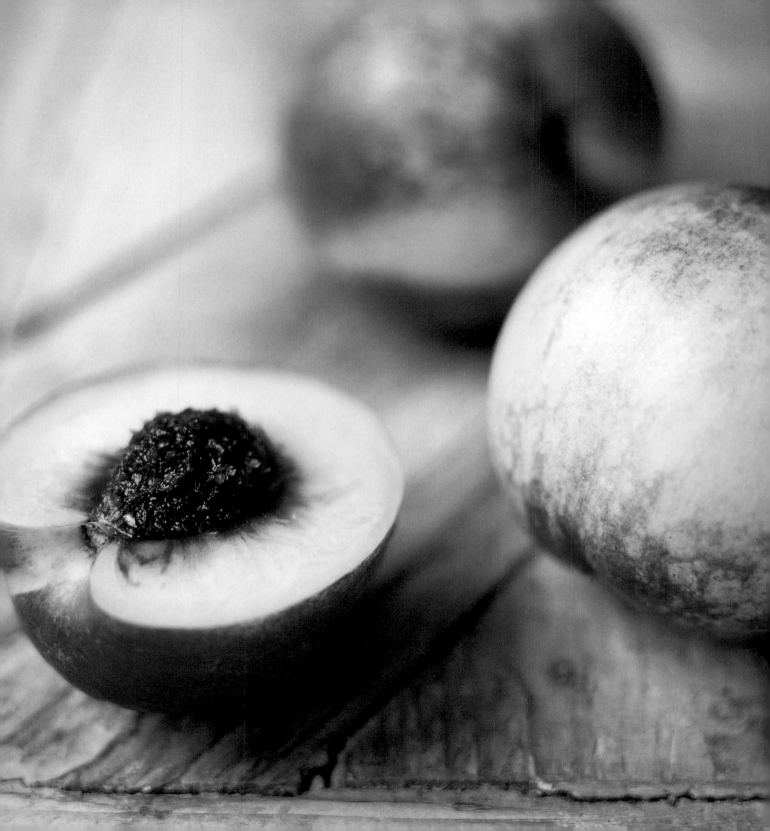

Putting it all together on your plate

It is important to start planning a meal by choosing a starchy carbohydrate as its basis. Then consider which fruit and vegetables would go well with it, and finally decide on a small portion of protein-rich food to balance the meal. For any given meal use the plate diagram below to help plan what you are going to eat.

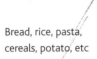

Bread, rice, pasta, cereals, potato, etc

Meat, fish, chicken, pulses, dairy

Fruits and vegetables

Half of your plateful should be in the form of starchy carbohydrates.

One-eighth of your plateful should consist of protein-rich food.

The rest should be made up of fruits and vegetables for the meal (remembering to eat five portions in total per day).

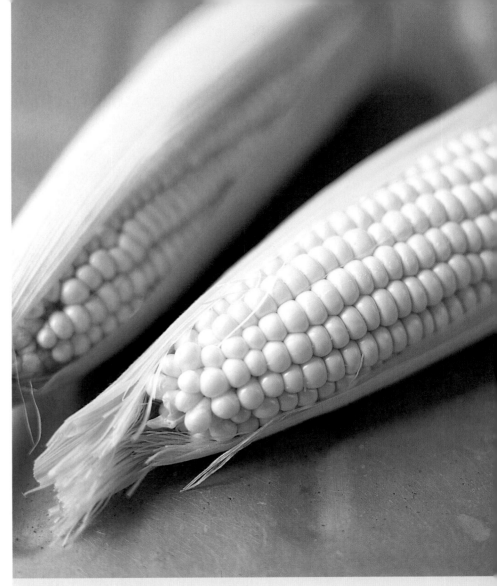

Simple meal plan using the plate method

	STARCHY/COMPLEX CARBOHYDRATE	PROTEIN OR DAIRY	FRUIT AND/OR VEGETABLES
Breakfast	Cereal	2% milk	Banana
Lunch	Wholewheat bread	Tuna	Cucumber and apple
Supper	Baked potato	Roast chicken, yogurt	Peas, corn, fruit salad

Portion sizes

Now that you know what to choose, you need to know how much to choose. As a guide, the list below shows the average portion sizes of basic food groups.

Average single serving/portion sizes
Starchy/complex carbohydrates
- 1 slice wholewheat bread
- ½ bread roll
- 4 small crackers
- 1 average bowl cereal
- 1 medium potato
- ½ cup cooked pasta, rice, etc.

Fruits and vegetables
- 1 medium fruit
- 2 small fruits
- ½ cup fruit juice
- 1 heaping tablespoon dried fruit
- ½ cup cooked vegetables
- ½ cup raw leafy vegetables

Protein group
- About 3½ oz. or pack of cards-size portion of red meat or chicken
- 2 thin slices ham
- 5oz. fish
- 1 cup cooked pulses
- ½ cup seeds or nuts

Dairy group
- 1 cup (9fl. oz.) milk or yogurt
- 1oz. or matchbox-size portion of cheese

Good eating habits

Often just by revisiting the following good, sensible, basic healthy eating practices you will soon start to notice an improvement in your symptoms.

Eating patterns

Try to eat three times a day every day, and if you need to snack, be sure to keep the snacks small, regular, and healthy. Regular dietary intake speeds up the metabolic rate, which enables you to burn calories more efficiently. The gut has also been seen to respond favorably to regular meal patterns.

Meal timing

Eat your meals at regular and normal times and try and keep these times consistent from day to day. Breakfast is best before 9 a.m., lunch between 12 and 2 p.m. and supper not later than 9 p.m. Do not skip meals.

Food volume

Eat approximately the same amount of food at each meal. Do not have small meals throughout the day and then indulge in a large meal at night. Concentrate on eating the same volume of food from meal to meal.

Eating atmosphere

Eat at a table in a relaxed atmosphere away from distractions and work. Turn the computer and television off and concentrate on what you are doing. Try to create a peaceful, relaxed, and calm environment. On working days, consider having your lunch in the park away from the distractions of an office.

Eating pace

Try to spend 20 minutes eating your meal—don't ever rush it. Think about chewing slowly, and put your knife and fork down between mouthfuls.

The role of fiber

Now that you have established a decent, healthy, balanced diet you will notice an improvement in your symptoms. To consolidate on this further you should next start to investigate the fiber content of your diet. First, a little insight into fiber and its role in the body.

What is fiber?

Fiber is the structural part of a plant, the framework that supports the plant and holds it together. It is therefore a component that is found only in foods of plant origin. It is part of the carbohydrate group, and often referred to as NSP (non-starch polysaccharide) in scientific circles or roughage in layman's terms. It is extremely hardy—you can chew it, swallow it, and subject it to stomach acids, yet most of it passes through your body unchanged.

Fiber acts in the bowel to:
- Regularize bowel function.
- Increase fecal weight.
- Improve the time it takes to move the stool through the colon.

There are many types of fiber, but from a dietary perspective we have two major classifications: soluble fiber and insoluble fiber. Plant foods mostly contain a combination of these two types and it is easiest to classify all fiber-containing foods according to which type is predominant. The latest thinking is that bowel function is most benefited by a combination of these two fiber types as they each have a different effect on the gut.

Soluble fiber

Food types which are predominantly high in soluble fiber are:
- Fruits
- Vegetables
- Legumes
- Oats
- Barley
- Seeds

Soluble fiber is effectively broken down by enzyme-producing bacteria present in the colon to produce energy and gas. If you eat too much soluble fiber the stools will be bulky, ribbon-like, and hard to pass. Soluble fiber contributes to an increase in bacterial mass of the stool. It forms a gel-like substance which can bind to other substances in the gut, having the additional benefits of lowering blood cholesterol levels and slowing down the entry of glucose into the blood, thereby improving blood sugar control.

Insoluble fiber

Foods predominantly high in insoluble fiber are:
- Roughage foods with skins, husks, and peels, e.g., spelt, buckwheat, millet, chickpeas
- Some fruit and vegetables with their skins and pits, e.g. tomatoes, zucchini, grapes, plus potatoes and other root vegetables
- Wheat, rye, and all other cereals
- Nuts and some legumes, e.g. almonds, chestnuts, coconut, chickpeas
- Rice

Insoluble fiber is less easily broken down by colonic bacteria than soluble fiber but holds water very effectively (up to 15 times its weight in water), thus contributing to an increase in stool weight and making the bowel work more efficiently. It is this fiber that is often referred to as "nature's broom" and it has been proved to have many protective effects in the gut against diseases like cancer, IBS, Crohn's disease, and others.

How much fiber do we need?

There is no simple answer to this question. Each person's fiber intake needs to be individually assessed and the contribution of the different fiber sources in their diet ascertained. This information serves then as a basis for dietary manipulation. It should be noted that there is a very fine line to be drawn between having the correct amount and overdoing it in terms of fiber intake. Prudent guidelines (that is, the recommended average for the population) suggest a total fiber intake of 20–30g (¾–1¼ oz.) per day of which one third needs to be soluble. A diet that contains a larger percentage of soluble fiber—that is, greater proportions of fruit, vegetables, and pulses to starchy carbohydrates—will perform very sluggishly. The stool will be soft, ribbon-like, and hard to pass as it contains no bulk to push against the bowel wall and make the muscle contract naturally. Correct fiber balance will fall into place naturally by following simple healthy eating rules using the plate method (see page 20). As long as you keep the proportions between the food groups right on your plate and stay within your specific fiber allowance, you will achieve a good balance of fiber types. It is important to remember that although these guidelines of 20–30g (¾–1¼ oz.) per day are prudent, they may not be appropriate for you. Your type of IBS and an assessment of your particular symptoms and present fiber intake will determine the amount of fiber that is right for you.

How much fiber do you have in your diet?

Have another look through your diet these past seven days and, using the fiber table on pages 24–25, assess which group your average fiber intake per day falls into:

Low   0–12g (0–½ oz.) per day
Medium   12–18g (½–¾ oz.) per day
High   18–25g (¾–1oz.) per day

How to achieve your optimum fiber intake

There are three different ways of manipulating your fiber intake, which can be summed up as follows.

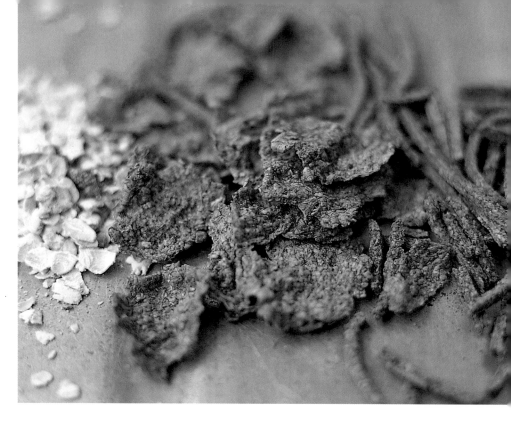

▶ **By following a healthy natural diet, with careful attention to the types and amount of fiber in foods.**
This option is undoubtedly the best. It will ensure that not only are your fiber sources natural and varied, but also that you can keep a careful control on the amount of fiber you are consuming, bearing in mind that different IBS patients need varying quantities. Your diet will also contain the correct balance of all other nutrients, ensuring a healthy, balanced, prudent intake.

▶ **By eating fiber-enriched foods.**
Foods such as specially produced high-fiber muffins and cookies or wheat-free, low-starch products will most certainly allow you to manipulate your fiber intake but will not rectify any other dietary imbalances. Such items are often too high in fat and sugar to be considered part of a healthy balanced diet.

▶ **By taking fiber extracts or supplements in the form of bran, pills, tablets, powders, and granules.**
Supervised use of bulk-forming laxatives can be beneficial in the early stages of dietary manipulation, but should not be viewed as a long-term solution. Some research has indicated that consistent use of one type of fiber, such as digestive bran, over a long period of time will result in it losing its effectiveness.

Fiber content of basic foods

FIBER CONTENT OF CEREALS, GRAINS, AND BREADS	PORTION SIZE	LOW (0–3g)	MEDIUM (3–5g)	HIGH (6g or more)
Breakfast cereals	**1 average bowl**			
Corn flakes	30g (1¼oz.)	0.3		
High-fiber bran cereal (e.g., All-Bran)	40g (1½oz.)			9.8
Muesli (no added sugar)	40g (1½oz.)		3	
Instant hot rolled oat cereal (e.g., Ready Brek)	160g (5½oz.)	2.2		
Puffed wheat (e.g., Sugar Puffs)	20g (¾oz.)	1.2		
Oatmeal (cooked)	160g (5½oz.)	1.3		
Bran flakes	30g (1¼oz.)		3.9	
Fruit and fiber	40g (1½oz.)	2.8		
Raisin Bran	40g (1½oz.)		4	
Toasted rice and wheat flakes (e.g., Special K)	30g (1¼oz.)	0.5		
Malted barley extract wholewheat cereal (e.g., Shreddies)	30g (1¼oz.)	2.3		
Wholegrain wheat cereal (e.g., Shredded Wheat)	2 pieces			6.1
Breads and biscuits				
White bread	2 medium slices	1		
Brown bread	2 medium slices	2.8		
Wholewheat bread	2 medium slices		4.5	
Wheatgerm bread	2 medium slices	2.6		
Hi-bran bread	2 medium slices			6.2
Pita bread (brown)	1 small (75g/3oz.)		3	
Granary bread	2 medium slices		3	
Rye bread	2 medium slices	2.6		
Graham crackers	1	0.4		
Rye crackers (e.g., Ryvita)	3 pieces		3.6	
Wheat crackers (e.g., wheat thins)	2 crackers		4.4	
Wholewheat crackers	3 crackers	1		
Pasta and rice				
White rice	180g (6oz.) cooked	0.2		
Brown rice	180g (6oz.) cooked	1.4		
White pasta	220g (8oz.) cooked	2.6		
Brown pasta	220g (8oz.) cooked			8
Barley	150g (5oz.) cooked		3	

FIBER CONTENT OF FRUIT, VEGETABLES, AND PULSES	PORTION SIZE	LOW (0–1.5g)	MEDIUM (1.6–3g)	HIGH (3g or more)
Fruit				
Apple (with peel)	1 medium (100g/4oz.)		1.8	
Apricots, dried	5 halves			3.4
Apricots, stewed	medium portion (50g/2oz.)	1.1		
Banana	1 medium (100g/4oz.)	1.1		
Dates, dried	1 (15g/½oz.)	0.6		
Figs, dried	1 (20g/¾oz.)	1.5		
Grapes	small bunch (100g/4oz.)	0.7		
Grapefruit	½ medium (80g/3oz.)	1		
Nectarine	1 medium (150g/5oz.)		1.7	
Melon	¼ slice (183g/6¼oz.)	1.3		
Peaches	1 medium (110g/4oz.)	1.4		
Oranges	1 medium (160g/5½oz.)		2.7	
Pears	1 medium (150g/5oz.)			3
Plums	1 medium (55g/2oz.)	0.9		
Prunes, dried	3		1.7	
Prunes, stewed	6	0.8		

FIBER CONTENT OF FRUIT, VEGETABLES, AND PULSES	PORTION SIZE	LOW (0–1.5g)	MEDIUM (1.6–3g)	HIGH (3g or more)
Raspberries, blackberries	medium portion (60g/2½ oz.)	1.5		
Red currants	medium portion (60g/2½ oz.)	1.5		
Cranberries	medium portion (75g/3oz.)		2.3	
Strawberries	medium portion (100g/4oz.)	1.1		
Golden raisins	1 tablespoon	0.6		
Raisins	1 tablespoon	0.6		
Black currants	140g (4½ oz.)			3.9
Gooseberries	140g (4½ oz.)		2.7	
Rhubarb	140g (4½ oz.)		1.7	
Vegetables (cooked)				
New potatoes	medium portion (175g/6oz.)		2.6	
Potatoes, old (no skin)	medium portion (180g/6oz.)		1.8	
Potatoes, jacket (with skin)	medium portion (180g/6oz.)			4.9
Brussels sprouts	medium portion (90g/3½ oz.)		2.4	
Fine beans	medium portion (90g/3½ oz.)			3.7
Peas	medium portion (70g/3oz.)			3.6
Eggplant	medium portion (80g/3oz.)	1.8		
Broccoli	medium portion (85g/3½ oz.)		2	
Carrots	medium portion (80g/3oz.)		2	
Spinach	medium portion (90g/3½ oz.)		1.9	
Tomatoes	medium portion (85g/3½ oz.)	0.9		
Corn	medium portion (85g/3½ oz.)	1.2		
Cabbage	medium portion (95g/3¾ oz.)		1.7	
Zucchini	medium portion (100g/4oz.)	1.2		
Leeks	medium portion (75g/3oz.)	1.3		
Parsnips	medium portion (65g/2½ oz.)			3
Salad/vegetables (raw)				
Bean sprouts	1 tablespoon	0.3		
Beets	1 portion (100g/4oz.)		1.9	
Cabbage	medium portion (90g/3½ oz.)		2.2	
Celery	1 stalk (30g/1¼ oz.)	0.4		
Cucumber	1 slice (6g/¼ oz.)	0.1		
Lettuce	1 portion (20g/¾ oz.)	0.2		
Mushrooms	1 medium (10g/½ oz.)	0.1		
Onions	1 medium (60g/2½ oz.)	0.8		
Scallions	1 bulb (10g/½ oz.)	0.2		
Peppers	1 slice (10g/½ oz.)	0.2		
Radishes	1 medium (8g/½ oz.)	0.1		
Tomatoes	1 medium (85g/3½ oz.)	0.9		
Legumes/pulses/nuts				
Aduki, kidney, navy, black-eyed beans (boiled)	medium portion (60g/2½ oz.)			3.3
Split peas, lentils (boiled)	medium portion (60g/2½ oz.)		1.6	
Baked beans	medium portion (135g/4½ oz.)			4.7
Borlotti, cannellini, lima beans	medium portion (60g/2½ oz.)		2.8	
Chickpeas (boiled)	medium portion (60g/2½ oz.)		2.6	
Almonds	25g (1oz.)	1.9		
Coconut	25g (1oz.)	1.8		
Hazelnuts	25g (1oz.)	1.6		
Peanuts	25g (1oz.)	1.6		
Brazil	25g (1oz.)	1.1		
Walnuts	25g (1oz.)	0.9		

Symptom-based Dietary Treatment of IBS

With a better understanding of how to eat a healthy balanced diet and of the science behind fiber, we can focus on your symptoms and show you how to manipulate your diet according to your bowel function by using fiber.

Most types of IBS will always be associated with crampy abdominal pain, sometimes relieved on defecation. Most patients will also experience abdominal fullness, gas, bloating, and swelling. Therefore we assess which group you fall into on a basis of your bowel movements. Are they:

▸ Constipation predominant?
▸ Diarrhea predominant?
▸ Alternating between constipation and diarrhea?

Use the recommendations for your type of IBS as set out below to work out how to manipulate your fiber intake. The recipes in this book are classified as being either low, medium or high fiber so that you can choose appropriate meals for your specific needs. See page 41 for more information on using the recipes.

The constipation-predominant sufferer

If this is you, you need more fiber in your diet. Having assessed your fiber intake, you now need to start increasing it gradually from low to high. Too rapid an increase will result in pain, cramping, and possibly even diarrhea, which will result in you losing confidence in the treatment and not carrying it through. Take it slowly and aim to increase your intake by just 5g (¼ oz.) fiber per day over a period of three to four weeks.

For example, if after assessing your diet you find that your basic fiber intake is just 10g (½ oz.) per day, for the next month you need to achieve 15g (⅔ oz.) per day, dividing it into 5g (¼ oz.) per meal. If after a month on this regime your symptoms are improving, you will need to increase your fiber intake again, this time to 20g (¾ oz.) per day (that is, about 6–7g/⅓ oz. per meal). Finally, after another month, you may need to push it up to 24g (1oz.) per day or 8g (⅓ oz.) fiber per meal. What you are looking to achieve is a regular, consistent, predictable bowel movement every day.

Choose your meals according to the healthy meal plate (see page 20) ensuring that the meal is based on complex carbohydrates (see page 18). This will result in a larger percentage of your fiber intake coming from insoluble fiber. Be sure to maintain regular meal times.

Take your total fiber allowance for the day and spread it out into three meals. Use the fiber table on pages 24–25 and the recipes in this book to ensure you are getting approximately the same amount of fiber at each meal. Aim ultimately to achieve 22–28g (¾–1¼ oz.) of fiber per day, depending on your tolerance. Adjust your dose of or wean yourself off any prescribed bulking agent or laxative as your fiber goal is reached.

Rotate your fiber food choices—do not get into the habit of eating the same foods week after week. Research with digestive bran has shown that we develop a type of immunity to one fiber type, so it is best to rotate your fiber choices as often as possible, ensuring a varied diet.

The diarrhea-predominant sufferer

For patients with ongoing diarrhea the first step is to decrease all fiber or residue in the diet to allow the bowel to rest and regenerate. The low-fiber/residue, low-fat diet (see the table opposite) is one that removes all fibrous substances as well as any food item that leaves residue behind after digestion. Plan your meals using the healthy meal plate, as illustrated on page 20, but stick to the foods on your allowed list. It is extremely difficult to ensure proper nutritional balance on such a restricted diet. Normally diarrhea ceases after two to three weeks on this diet. If it doesn't you should seek a dietitian's advice to ensure it is safe to continue with the diet and that you are carefully monitored so that no unnecessary deficiencies arise. If the diarrhea doesn't stop, you may need to start a supervised exclusion diet (see page 31).

You should take a good multivitamin while you are on the low-fiber/residue diet, along with a good-quality probiotic supplement in order to replace lost gut-friendly bacteria.

After two or three weeks if the diarrhea has settled down, you can start reintroducing fiber to your meals. Be cautious as your bowel will be very sensitive and will need a very slow

The low-fiber/residue, low-fat diet

FOODS ALLOWED	FOODS TO AVOID
White flour and flour products, e.g., white bread, wafer cookies, plain sponge cake, sandwich cake, plain crackers	Brown bread and all wholewheat flour products, wholewheat crispbreads, Graham crackers, and other crackers and cookies, fruit cake, fruit desserts, oat cakes
Toasted rice cereal (e.g., Rice Krispies), corn flakes, cooked and strained oatmeal	Bran cereals, wholegrain wheat cereal (e.g., Shredded Wheat), wheat crackers (e.g., wheat thins), rolled oats, and granola
White rice and pasta	Brown rice and wholewheat pasta
Fruit juices Stewed or strained fruit Tender whole canned fruit	Fresh fruit with skins, pits, or seeds All dried fruits
Soft baby carrots Well-cooked vegetables	All raw vegetables, salads, pulses
Clear and well-puréed light soups	Vegetable soups
Peeled potatoes—mashed or boiled	Potatoes with skins—fried, roast, baked
Lean, tender meat and poultry	Fried and highly seasoned meats, duck, goose, meat products e.g., sausages and meat pies
Boneless fish—broiled or poached	Fried, oily, bony fish, e.g., herring, trout, kippers, sardines
1 cup low-fat milk per day OR ½ cup low-fat milk and 1 small low-fat yogurt Small amounts of regular cheese Eggs Butter and other fats in moderation	Cream, fruit yogurt Fried eggs
Jello and sorbet	Fruit desserts, ice cream
Sugar, jellies and marmalade, honey, syrup	Coarse marmalade, jellies with pits or skins
Salt	Pepper, pickles, strongly flavored spices
Squashes, carbonated drinks	Strong tea and coffee

reacquaintance with fiber. Add one new item at a time, distributing the fiber evenly throughout the day within fiber types and meals. IBS patients in this group tend to settle on a lower amount of fiber (18g/¾ oz.) than the constipation-predominant types.

The alternating diarrhea and constipation sufferer

If your symptoms alternate between diarrhea and constipation, you should approach fiber manipulation in the same way as described for the constipation-predominant sufferer, taking careful note of your symptoms at each step.

If your diarrhea worsens after slowly increasing your fiber as described above, decrease your fiber intake to under 10g (½ oz.) per day for two to four weeks. If things settle down, gradually start increasing it again; then, if there still is no change in your symptoms, consider the non-dietary aspects of your treatment, such as stress management and lifestyle changes.

Try to get all aspects of the treatment in place before making a judgment on how effective the diet is. You may be following the most perfect diet but find that a lack of fluid or a stressful event can cause your symptoms to be the same as before or worse. In other words, get your house in order before judging the effect of the diet.

If everything is in place but symptoms are persisting, it may mean that you need to start the exclusion diet (see page 31).

Gas and bloating

Often IBS sufferers find that once their bowel function is back to normal they are still left with some gas, bloating, and sometimes abdominal cramps. There are a number of treatment solutions depending on the cause, the most common of which are outlined below.

1. Too much fiber too soon (that is, more than 30g (1⅓ oz.) per day)

IBS sufferers who are eager to see improvement (understandably) will often get going with their new high-fiber diet a little too enthusiastically. If you are not used to fiber in your gut, it is best to start introducing it slowly, increasing it by 5g (¼ oz.) every four weeks. Sometimes patients return a month later to their doctor for a follow-up visit, full of complaints about experiencing worse symptoms of gas and bloating than they started with. Their immediate assumption is that they must have an intolerance to wheat. On analysis of their food diary it is often obvious that they have far exceeded their fiber prescription and in a very short space of time have even tripled their fiber intake.

The lazy bowel which is not used to fiber tends to react badly to too much too soon. Experience shows that a slow but consistent reintroduction of fiber to a fiber-depleted diet is the most successful course. Small increments of 5g (¼ oz.) extra fiber per month seem best tolerated. The solution in such cases is either to cut back immediately to a more manageable level of fiber intake, wait until symptoms dissipate and then slowly try to increase your intake of total fiber again, balancing up the fiber types and distribution among meals. Some patients complain that this initial process of building up their fiber intake leaves them with not enough to eat. In such cases try taking in extra food in the form of low-fat refined carbohydrates such as plain cookies, white bread, and crackers.

2. Too much total fiber (that is, more than 30g (1⅓ oz.) per day)

There are those who are so eager to increase their fiber intake that they take it way over the top limit of 30g (1⅓ oz.) per day without realizing it. There seems to be a very fine line between having too little and too much fiber and the latter can cause excessive bowel movement, bloating, and gas. If you have fallen into this trap, decrease your total fiber to a level that is comfortable to produce the best and most satisfying bowel habit.

3. Too much soluble fiber

A high intake of soluble versus insoluble fiber can also lead to excess amounts of food residues available for gut fermentation in the colon. Soluble fiber is metabolized by healthy gut bacteria to produce short-chain fatty acids (energy) and gases. In certain people who harbor excessive amounts of sulphur-producing bacteria, extra gases such as hydrogen sulphide and methanethiol are also produced, which result in bad smelly gas. The short-chain fatty acids feed the colonic bacteria, increasing their quantity and fermentation rate and so producing an increase in bowel gases.

It is a common error, when attempting to increase your fiber intake, to be over-enthusiastic and eat too great a quantity of fruits, vegetables, pulses, nuts, and seeds, which are the main sources of soluble fiber in our diet. In order to achieve the right balance, aim to maintain but not exceed the recommended five portions of fruit and vegetables per day and ensure that all starch portions in your meals are those which contain insoluble fiber. Do not make the mistake of counting oats as an insoluble source when they are actually classified as a soluble fiber (see page 22). Be aware, too, of the perils of the smoothie revolution. Smoothies are healthy drinks in that they do contain massive amounts of vitamins, but they also contribute a large load of soluble fiber which you don't necessarily need.

4. Bacterial overgrowth

Bacterial overgrowth can occur as a result of an excessive intake of soluble fiber, as discussed above, resulting in an increase in the number of bacteria in the bowel and subsequent increases in colonic gas production.

Moreover, the value of probiotics (see page 34) for the IBS patient has not yet been clearly established. They have been shown to benefit sufferers from post-infective type IBS, but for the time being we still need to be conscious that too much of a "good" thing can also be bad. If we load our bowel with excesses of these good bacteria, are we not supplying more bacteria to ferment available food residues and so produce even more gas?

5. "Gassy" foods

Certain foods, particularly those from the brassica plant family (such as cabbages and Brussels sprouts) are notorious for producing gassy bowels, probably due to the sulphur-containing compounds found in many of them. A very basic list of other possible culprit foods is given below. There is no need to avoid them all; instead, keep the list on the fridge and when you experience a very bad bout of abdominal gas, check the list to see if you have eaten any of these foods.

Foods and drinks that have been associated with an increased production of intestinal gas

Fish	Asparagus
Milk products	Garlic
Dried beans	Sweet potatoes
Cucumbers	Corn
Mushrooms	Yeast
Onions	Melons
Brussels sprouts	Nuts
Peas	Sugar
Spinach	Candies
Cabbage	
Broccoli	Carbonated drinks
Radishes	Sweetened drinks
Cauliflower	Beer

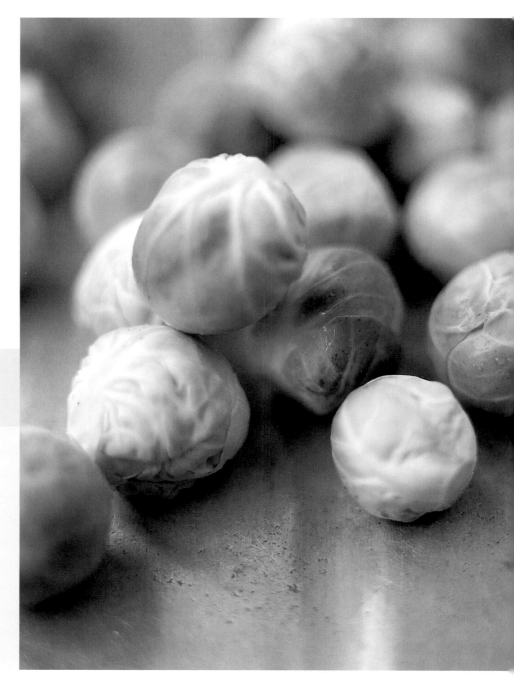

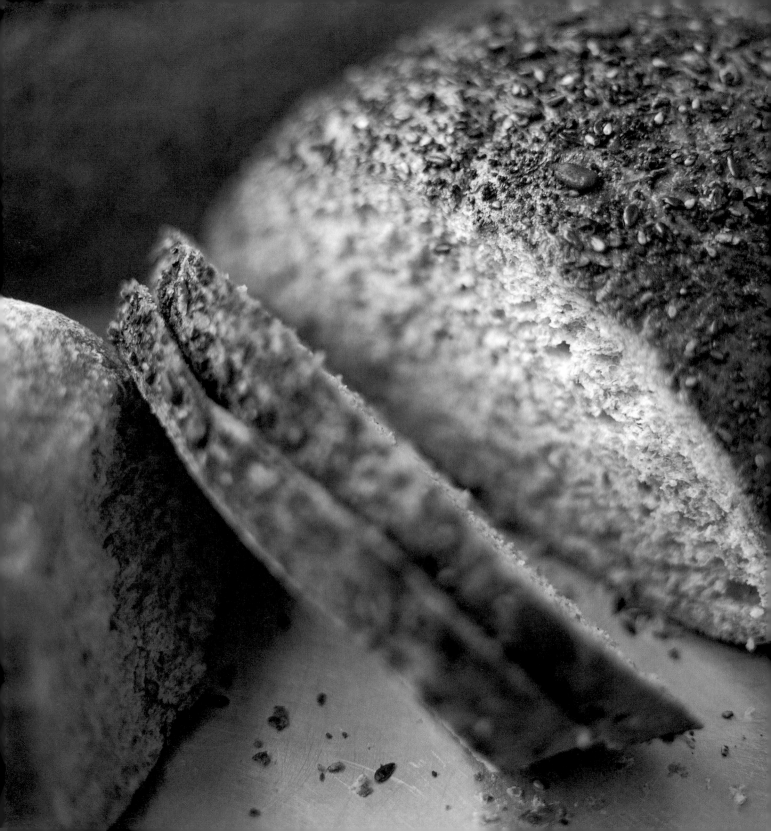

Practical tips to increase your fiber intake

▶ Ensure that all the starch or grains that you eat are the high-fiber varieties. Read the labels of breakfast cereals and breads to check.

▶ Switch to whole grain breads (which should contain at least 2–3g of fiber per slice).

▶ Introduce more whole grains, such as wholewheat pasta and brown rice, into your main meal.

▶ Have three servings of fruit and two of vegetables per day, where possible raw and with their skins, pits, and membranes. Start the day by including a piece of fresh fruit in your breakfast, have fruit as a dessert in your main meal and as a between-meal snack.

▶ Don't forget the fluid. Without fluid, dietary fiber cannot do its job. Drink at least 6–8 cups per day. Suitable fluids include all non-caffeine and non-alcohol-based fluids like water, herbal teas, and well-diluted fruit juices.

▶ If you need to snack, choose high-fiber options, such as dried fruit, nuts and raisins, wholewheat crackers and rusks, popcorn.

▶ Try to include cooked beans, peas or lentils as part of your main meal.

▶ Avoid processed, preprepared foods: they have a lower fiber content than their fresh alternatives.

Food intolerance and food exclusion

From the above dietary prescriptions and comments you will note that eliminating any item of food from your diet should be the absolute last resort. All too often patients eliminate important nutrients without fully investigating the causes of their actions. True food allergy/intolerance is in fact very rare. Many people end up developing what we refer to as a perceived food intolerance, where their brain-gut axis is very much involved, and although these people do not have a real intolerance, because of what they have read and how certain circumstances have evolved, they react as if they are actually intolerant. It is a challenge for the doctors and dietitians involved in their care to gain their trust to try these eliminated food items again.

Foods which seem most likely to cause true allergenic reactions are dairy products, coffee, wheat, eggs, corn, potatoes, onions, citrus fruit, and yeasts. An exclusion diet involves eating only a few foods or a low allergenic diet for a few weeks and then slowly introducing one new food at a time, taking careful note of your symptoms along the way. It is a long, drawn-out process that often reveals quite inconclusive results.

Any attempt to eliminate these "suspect" foods from your diet should be done only under supervision by a state-registered dietitian when all other avenues of IBS treatment have been exhausted.

Weight gain and the high-fiber diet

Maintaining and/or losing weight are major concerns for many of us. Often, when people are faced with the concept of eating more carbohydrate, panic sets in. The reason is that when eating this way you will find that you are consuming larger volumes of food. Complex carbohydrates are bulky and it seems bigger on your plate. The aim is to achieve a bulkier diet to get your bowels moving more consistently. However, high-fiber foods, provided they are prepared in a healthy low-fat manner, will not increase your calorie intake, and some people, who up to now have been eating a high-fat diet, will see their calorie intake actually decrease. Rest assured that this way of eating will make your bowel function better and could even result in some weight loss.

What About Fluid?

We are all aware that we need to drink suitable amounts of fluid, but how vital is it and how many of us actually do it? Taking too little of the right fluid and too much of the wrong fluid can be disastrous for your health. It is all too easy to let the whole day pass without having enough fluid.

The human body is made up on average of 50 percent water. If you are an athlete, this can go up to 60 percent. If you are overweight, the figure drops to around 40 percent. This is because lean muscle tissue contains more water than fat tissue. About two-thirds of the water in the body is contained in cells; the other third travels around the body in blood and body fluids. In an average male this third can be equivalent to 3 gallons of fluid.

A normal healthy person loses water all the time through evaporation from the skin, lungs, urine, and feces. Lost volumes can total up to 4½ pints per day, so provision of sufficient fluids ensures an optimal internal environment for regulating digestion, absorption, metabolism, and excretion. A loss or decrease in body fluids lessens the efficiency of the mechanisms at work within your body, preventing the major organs from working at their most efficient rate.

Continuous mild dehydration can also result in:

▶ Constipation. Fluid is vital for softening the fiber eaten in order to prevent constipation. Too little fluid will result in hard stools that are difficult to pass. Without fluid, dietary fiber cannot do its job. Insoluble fiber in particular acts like a sponge absorbing water, increasing stool weight and size, thus putting pressure on the bowel wall and facilitating movement of the stool. Without fluid this fiber is pointless and will only constipate you further.

▶ Cystitis. Too little fluid provides an environment in the bladder that encourages unhealthy bacteria. Increased fluid intake will provide a healthy flow through the bladder, preventing any accumulation of unhealthy bacteria.

▶ Dehydration. Symptoms of lethargy, headaches, and generally feeling off color are signs of mild dehydration, though not easily recognized as such. Excessive alcohol intake can also lead to dehydration.

When fluid is lost from your body, the concentration of salt in the blood rises, causing the mechanism of thirst to be activated. However, don't assume that you are drinking enough just because you are not thirsty. As we get older our ability to detect thirst diminishes.

We can obtain water for our bodies from both the fluid we drink and the food we eat. Although the recommendation is to drink 6–8 cups per day, this is only a guideline and fluid needs are rather individual. They depend on your body size and structure, level of fitness and dietary factors such as your caffeine and alcohol intake.

The best monitor is the color of your urine and the frequency of urination. Urine that is pale yellow and frequent is a good sign that plenty of fluid is available for waste excretion. Bright yellow urine is an indication of a dehydrated body. (Note, however, that vitamin B supplementation can cause urine to become dark yellow in color.)

What to drink?
Water and watery drinks

Water is the best option. You may wish to drink bottled spring or mineral water, still or sparkling. Have what you like best, because that will ensure you drink the biggest volume. There is nothing wrong with tap water, and in many cases tap water is subject to more regulations regarding purity than bottled water. Some bottled water is fortified with minerals such as calcium and magnesium. If you live in a hard-water area, check the mineral content of your tap water with your supplier—you may be surprised to learn that it has a higher mineral content than that of bottled water.

Fruit juice comes next, but dilute them to the maximum as their sugar content can be high.

Try also herbal and fruit teas, but be wary of green teas as most varieties are rather high in caffeine.

Keep carbonated drinks to a minimum (not more than one a day) as they are high in sugar and additives.

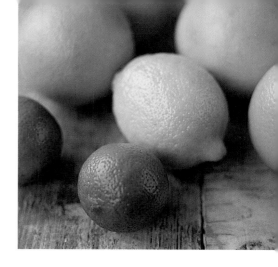

Caffeine

Most of us eat caffeine-rich foods such as chocolate and drink caffeine-rich fluids. Caffeine stimulates the heart and central nervous system and acts within our bodies in the same way as amphetamines, cocaine, and heroin. It is therefore addictive and dehydrating. If you feel you cannot function without it, you are addicted to caffeine. Some people consume up to 1000mg per day, equivalent to ten cups of percolated coffee or 15 cups of instant coffee. How much do you drink? Try to limit your intake of caffeine-rich fluids to no more than three drinks per day.

Alcohol

Be sensible about your alcohol consumption. Remember that alcohol has a diuretic effect, thus promoting an increase in normal fluid losses. In order for the body to process the dehydrating effects of one glass of wine, it will need the equivalent in water over and above your normal fluid intake. Don't forget that alcohol is very calorie-dense but nutrient-deficient, so replacing meals with alcohol on too many occasions can lead to nutritional deficiencies.

Sensible alcohol intakes

Men: 3–4 units per day or less
Women: 2–3 units per day or less
Have three alcohol-free days a week

1 unit =
½ pint of beer or
1 small glass of sherry or
1 small glass of wine or
1 single measure of spirits

Good alcohol habits to create

▶ Eat first, then drink alcohol.
▶ Alternate water and alcohol.
▶ Try low-alcohol or non-alcoholic drinks.
▶ Add low-calorie mixers to extend your drinks.
▶ Drink slowly, take small sips and pace yourself.
▶ After a bad drinking binge, give your body a 48-hour rest.

Good reasons to increase your fluid intake:
▶ Gets your body in motion.
▶ Avoids constipation.
▶ Increases nutrient absorption.
▶ Moisturizes your skin.
▶ Keeps your kidneys healthy.
▶ Decreases muscle cramps.
▶ Prevents kidney stones.
▶ Avoids dehydration.
▶ Regulates your body temperature.

Tips to help you drink more:
▶ Start drinking early in the day.
▶ Drink small amounts throughout the day.
▶ Have a bottle of water on your desk, in your car, and in your briefcase.
▶ Drink while traveling.
▶ Drink while exercising.
▶ Decrease the amount of tea, coffee, and alcohol you drink, create a thirst and replace it with water.
▶ Put a reminder on the screensaver on your computer.
▶ Try warm water.
▶ Try flavoring water with slices of fresh fruit.

Caffeine content of what you drink and eat	
Coffee mg per 7oz. cup	
Instant	61–70
Percolated	97–125
Tea mg per 7oz. cup	15–75
Cocoa mg per 7oz. cup	10–17
Chocolate (per 2½oz. milk chocolate)	60–70
Cola drinks mg per 11oz. can	43–65
Some sports drinks mg per 11oz. can	18
Performance Alert drinks mg per 8oz. can	75

The Alternative Side

Probiotics, prebiotics, and symbiotics

Recently there has been a flood of "fermented" or "live" products on our supermarket shelves, most of these based on dairy products. The processes of regulating our gut bacteria can be defined as three separate approaches:

▶ Probiotics
▶ Prebiotics
▶ Symbiotics

Probiotics are live microbial food supplements, widely used in "live" yogurts and dairy products. Best known are the lactic acid bacteria and bifidobacteria.

More recently and not as extensively marketed or researched are another group of foodstuffs known as the prebiotics. These are defined as non-digestible foodstuffs which pass through the bowel, arriving in the colon undigested. Here they are said to be selectively able to stimulate the growth of the above-mentioned probiotics. The group of carbohydrates called the oligosaccharides (a type of dietary fiber) is the best known of these.

This brings us to symbiotics, the third possibility of gut bacteria management. This involves the proposed interaction between certain probiotics and prebiotics in order to improve the survival of the probiotic and thus prolong its said benefits.

"Live" products promise to boost the body's natural resistance, promote healthy digestion, and improve the balance of our own gut microflora through the addition of probiotic bacteria. There is little, but growing, hard scientific evidence investigating the mechanisms and processes involved in this probiotic phenomenon. Indeed, probiotics do have a significant potential for improving human health and preventing and treating disease. Probiotic supplementation has, however, been seen to be beneficial in treating those with post-infective IBS by replacing valuable gut bacteria.

Lactose intolerance

One of the most common groups of foods avoided by IBS sufferers is milk and other dairy products. In a desperate attempt to find their own solution some IBS patients start eliminating lactose from their diet. When we adopt such a course of action, unfortunately we are often doing more harm than good.

What we do know is that lactose malabsorption may induce symptoms indistinguishable from certain variants of IBS, particularly the diarrhea-predominant type, such as nausea, abdominal discomfort, cramps, bloating, and diarrhea. These symptoms in lactose intolerance are brought about by fermentation of lactose in the intestine. It is easily seen how the two conditions can be confused and therefore it is strongly recommended that lactose malabsorption be properly excluded by your doctor before the diagnosis of IBS is made.

There is, however, a certain percentage of IBS patients who do have true lactose intolerance. The available research is very varied in terms of its conclusiveness as to the real incidence in IBS patients, but it does seem certain that some may well be lactose intolerant. It is just not nearly as many of you as you think. The best advice is not to self-diagnose. If you suspect that you may be intolerant to dairy products, seek your answer from the professionals. A physician will run a lactose-tolerance test, and if a positive diagnosis is made, it will be followed up with an appointment with a qualified dietitian to ensure that what needs to be eliminated from your diet will be replaced with suitable substitutes.

Sorbitol

Sorbitol is an artificial sweetener used in diet foods, soft drinks, and diabetic foods. Large doses of sorbitol or fructose-sorbitol mixtures have been seen to worsen or induce diarrhea in adults.

Peppermint

Peppermint is a natural antispasmodic that relaxes the muscles lining the bowel wall. Many doctors prescribe it as a first line of treatment. Study results have not been consistently positive, but if you would like to try peppermint, be sure to use enteric-coated capsules, which will only dissolve lower down in the gut and will not cause or aggravate heartburn. Peppermint tea has a milder effect than tablets.

Aloe vera

In some cases patients have reported that aloe vera has been beneficial in reducing IBS symptoms. Although there is no clear evidence to support its use, anecdotal evidence does suggest that aloe vera may ease discomfort by an anti-inflammatory and possibly immune-enhancing effect. It is available from health food stores and is most often taken in liquid form by adding 2 teaspoons to a glass of water.

Vegetarianism and IBS

Many vegetarians are not following a healthy balanced vegetarian diet. They have eliminated certain protein foods for whatever reason and not replaced them with suitable substitutes, resulting in a poorly balanced diet. However a carefully planned vegetarian diet generally corresponds very closely to healthy eating ideals in terms of fat, carbohydrate, and fiber content. This type of diet tends to be low in saturated fat, cholesterol, and animal protein and contains increasing concentrations of folate, antioxidants (vitamins C and E, carotinoids, and phytochemicals), and complex carbohydrates and fiber, all of which offer certain disease protection. Epidemiological studies have shown that vegetarians have a lower body weight, lower blood fat levels, and therefore decreased incidence of coronary heart disease.

Vegetarians also suffer from less hypertension (high blood pressure) and a lower risk of the complications arising from diabetes. This is perhaps due to their increased intake of fiber-rich foods and decreased body mass index (weight to height ratio). The incidence of lung, breast, and colon cancer is also less in vegetarians. It has been seen that the colon of a vegetarian differs greatly from that of a non-vegetarian and of course this definitely should have implications for the IBS patient.

Most vegetarian diets have a fiber intake that meets or exceeds the recommended dietary allowance (RDA) of 24g. The very fine line between having too much and too little fiber was explained earlier in this book. It is also important to ensure that you get the fiber ratio right, the largest percentage of your fiber intake coming from insoluble sources (such as cereals, breads, rice, pasta, and so on). In the vegetarian diet there is the advantage that the diet is naturally high in fiber, but can easily be too high, especially in soluble fiber (found in fruit, vegetables, pulses, and nuts). This will result in a worsening of IBS symptoms, with added bloating, gas, abdominal pain, and possibly diarrhea.

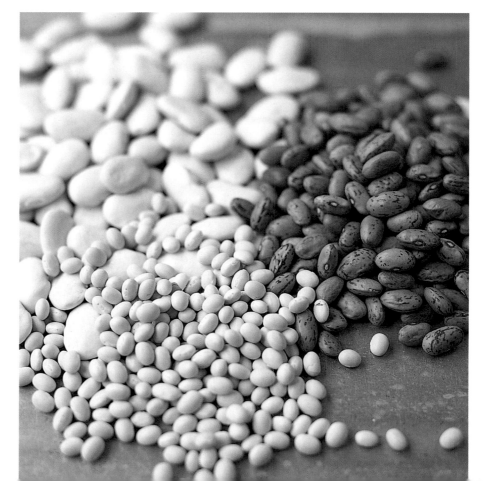

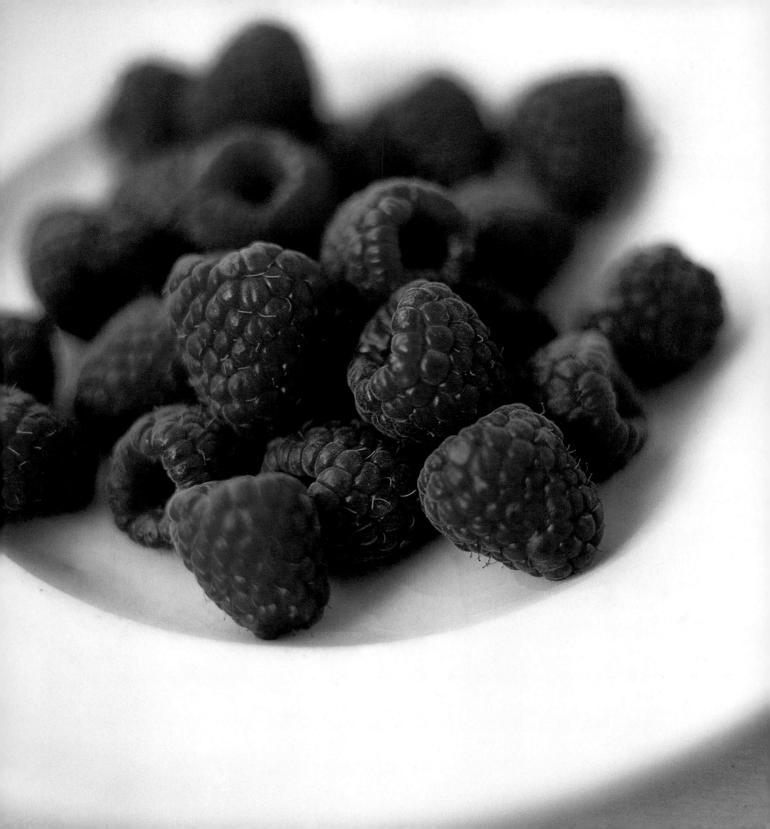

Shopping and Eating Out

Changing to this way of eating might mean a whole new way of shopping. We all tend to charge through the supermarket at a rapid pace, grabbing those same old things we always buy, so you will need to put a little time aside to cruise the aisles and stock up on some good high-fiber essential ingredients. Before you do that, you need to know what to choose and how to read labels.

Reading labels

We are lucky that food labeling is so well regulated these days. If you can understand what you are reading, this information is very useful in helping you plan your diet.

First, ingredients are listed in order of their weight content in that particular food, with the largest at the beginning. This information can be of use to people allergic to or avoiding certain foods—for example, sugars or gluten-containing products.

The nutritional content of a product is what an IBS patient really needs to look at. The most commonly listed nutrients are calories, protein, carbohydrates, sugar, fat (including saturates), fiber, and sodium. Nutrients are usually listed per manufacturer's recommended portion size of the product. It is important to check if you are eating the same portion size; if not, you will have to recalculate to get an accurate idea of what you are consuming.

The recommended daily values are designed to help you, the consumer, calculate how that given product would fit into a normal healthy diet for an adult of normal body weight. These are shown in the table to the right. So if you are choosing a product that is high in fat, perhaps a cheesy pasta dish, that uses up half your fat allowance for the day, you will be able to calculate how much fat you have "left" and know to choose lower-fat options from then on. Remember: these are meant only as a guideline, since needs vary from one person to another.

The "little and a lot" table, also shown above, has been devised to help you judge how much of a particular ingredient a food contains. It is useful when comparing one product with another and will help you determine if what you are buying is high enough in fiber and low enough in fat to meet your dietary requirements.

Choosing fresh foods

Obviously you need plenty of fresh fruit and vegetables. Use your lists and choose lots of high-fiber fruit and vegetables such as pears, oranges, apples, berries, spinach, broccoli, carrots, sprouts, corn, and so on. Vary your choice from store to store, and try things you don't normally buy.

Visit the bakery and get some freshly baked wholewheat grainy bread, then add some wholewheat pita bread, pumpernickel, and wholewheat muffins to your shopping basket. If you are following a low-fiber diet, go for refined, soft white breads.

Nutritional guidelines

A LOT	A LITTLE
20g fat	3g fat
5g saturates	1g saturates
3g fiber	0.5g fiber
10g sugars	2g sugars
0.5g sodium	0.1g sodium

If you want to know the amount of salt (sodium chloride) in a product, multiply the sodium by 2.5.

Recommended daily values

	MEN	WOMEN
Calories	2500 Calories	2000 Calories
Fat	80g	70g
Saturates	25g	20g
Fiber	30g	16g
Total Carb	375g	300g
Sodium	2400mg	2400mg

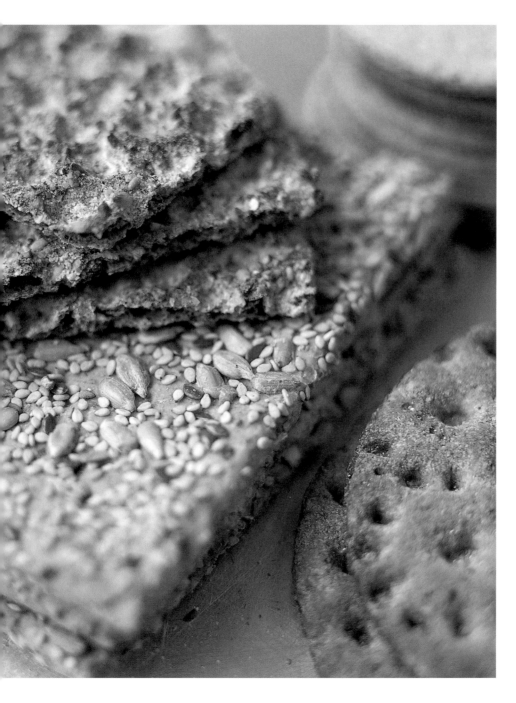

Choosing dry goods

Cereals and grains

Supermarket shelves are stocked with a wide range of high-fiber cereals. Read the labels and choose those that are low in fat and sugar but that meet your fiber requirements. Breakfast cereals are versatile in that they can be used in baked goods, as toppings or bases, or as an extender in meat dishes like meatballs. Wheat bran and rice bran are good sources of fiber to keep on hand to add to baked goods, desserts, and cereals to boost the insoluble fiber content.

Pulses

Buy dried beans, peas, lentils, chickpeas and so on in their dried or canned form. Canned pulses are easier to use as there is no need to soak and boil them—just open the can, rinse in water and add them to salads, vegetables, meat dishes, and soups.

Rice and pasta

Try brown rice, wild rice, red rice, and brown basmati rice, which all contain considerably more fiber than white rice.

Wholewheat pasta is a really good source of insoluble fiber, but it may contain too much fiber for your specific requirement, in which case mix it with white pasta to get used to the flavor and to build up your fiber intake. Spelt or faro pasta, which is used in some of the recipes in this book, is an excellent source of fiber and people often find it more acceptable in taste than the really nutty wholewheat pastas.

Cookies and crackers

Choose wholewheat, oat, and rye-based crackers and cookies, which are excellent for snacking on. Also keep a supply of Graham cracker-type biscuits for that sweet-tooth moment.

Dried fruit, nuts, and seeds

Keep a good variety of dried fruits, nuts, and seeds at home and at work. They are excellent snack foods as a very small quantity will contribute significant amounts of soluble fiber to your diet. They can also be easily added to vegetable dishes, used as a coating, and added to salads, desserts, and breakfast cereals when you have run out of fresh fruit.

Eating out

It is unreasonable to assume that you won't occasionally want fast foods or a nice meal in a restaurant. Don't avoid eating out because of this diet: it has to fit in with your lifestyle and life has to go on. Remember that when your eating plan is established, as long as you keep to it most of the time, the odd meal where you disregard the rules is not going to make that much of a difference to your symptoms. In time you will also find a few favorite restaurants where you know you can get a delicious meal that also meets your dietary requirements. It is possible to get sufficient amounts of fiber in some restaurants (such as French-style, Mexican, Eastern, English-style pubs, steak houses, or Italian). In others (Indian and burger shops) it is not that easy.

Quick tips for eating out

▶ If you will be eating in a restaurant where you know you will not get all the components required in your diet, a good way of taking the pressure off yourself (and to make sure that you enjoy the outing more) is to have a decent high-fiber snack before you go out—for example two rye crispbreads, a pear, a handful of nuts or some dried fruit. Then, at the restaurant, skip the starch option and just have the meat, fish, or chicken and the vegetables.

▶ Alternatively take some wholewheat or brown bread from the basket and have that instead of the low-fiber rice that may be offered.

▶ Always make sure you get some extra vegetables and/or salad with your main course.

▶ Choose the lowest-fat option that you can.

▶ Choose fruity desserts.

▶ If you drink wine or other alcohol, drink double the amount of water as well.

▶ Try not to overeat, even if the food tastes good.

▶ Try not to eat out too late in the evening.

French

Although sometimes served in smaller portions than you may be used to, this type of eating is in most cases reasonably healthy in terms of fat content but often rather lacking in insoluble-fiber options. It may be better to have your starch for the evening before you go out, in the form of a high-fiber cracker-type snack, then when you are at the restaurant you can concentrate on the beautifully prepared vegetables and protein dishes.

Mexican

The pulse content of Mexican meals makes them worthwhile for people on a high-fiber diet. Be wary, though, of the fat content of some menu items such as enchiladas, guacamole, sour cream, and fried tortillas. Rather, go for fajitas, vegetable dishes or bean, chickpea, and pulse dishes. Stay away from anything too spicy: it will aggravate the lining of your bowel wall and could worsen your symptoms.

Eastern

Here the noodles are a slightly better choice than the rice dishes, as they contain more fiber, but stick to the boiled and steamed options (not the fried noodles) for keeping your fat intake down. Vegetables, nuts, and seeds are plentiful in this type of cooking for good soluble-fiber content. Choose wisely to keep your fat down and your fiber up. Be cautious of the spicy dishes if these tend to worsen your symptoms.

English-style pub meals

Try a baked potato with a low-fat sauce like bolognaise, tuna, or perhaps some baked beans if you are looking for more fiber. Broiled fish with new potatoes and the vegetables of the day is a good option, or try a salad combined with some chunky high-fiber bread (watch out for the dressing, though).

Steak houses

This steak meal is quite a good choice mainly because you can control it all. You can order the size steak you want and choose your accompaniments, such as baked or new potatoes. Steak portions tend to be large but try to stick to 4½–5oz. maximum. Salads are normally available from a salad bar, which is just perfect for allowing you to control what you get. So you can end up with a really well-balanced meal that is high in fiber.

Italian

Choose pasta in preference to pizza—it has a fiber content worth counting, and is not nearly as high in fat as the average pizza. Also remember to go for tomato-based vegetable sauces rather than the creamy, cheesy, high-fat ones. Have a salad to start, with dressing on the side so that you can control the amount added.

Indian

It is hard to get suitable fiber in an Indian restaurant—rice, poppadums, and meat curries will not satisfy your fiber needs. You could go for the lentil, pulse-based, and vegetable curries, which will give you some soluble fiber. Perhaps have very little of the starch and fill up with a few high-fiber crackers when you get home. You will need to go for mildly flavored dishes rather than anything too hot and spicy. What tastes good now could cause irritation to your bowel tomorrow. Keep the fat down by choosing dry curries and tomato-based sauces like jalfrezi and rogan josh.

Fast food

Burgers and fried chicken are no good in any format, so don't go there.

Fish and chips are full of fat, and the only way you could get (soluble) fiber would be to have some baked beans or mushy peas with them.

Other takeout meals are covered by the information on various types of cuisine given above and on page 39.

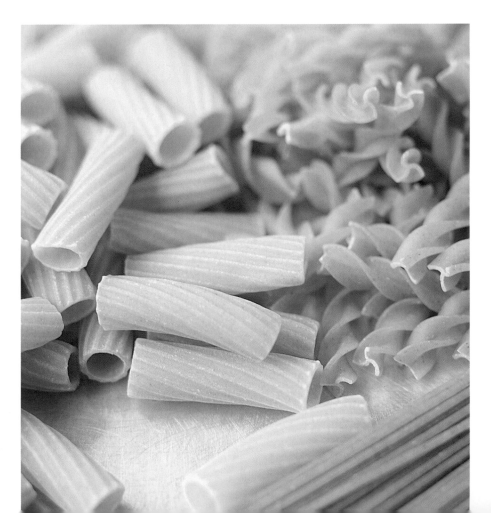

How to Use This Book

As we have seen, IBS is a complex condition and many factors are involved. We know that the best results in treatment are achieved when all aspects of the treatment are dealt with. Take some time to make sure you understand all the issues discussed so far, and put the following points into practice:

▶ Address lifestyle factors such as stress, relaxation, and exercise.
▶ Assess your current diet.
▶ Ensure you are meeting healthy eating guidelines.
▶ Put good eating habits into place.
▶ Ensure you are drinking enough fluids.

Once these factors are in place, you can determine the amount of fiber that is right for you by identifying which type of IBS you have and how much fiber you currently have in your diet. You will have already determined whether you have low, medium, or high levels of fiber in your diet as follows (see page 23):

Low	0–12g (0–½ oz.) per day
Medium	12–18g (½–¾ oz.) per day
High	18–25g (¾–1oz.) per day

You will also have decided which of the following best describes your bowel function:

▶ Constipation-predominant sufferer
▶ Diarrhea-predominant sufferer
▶ Alternating constipation and diarrhea sufferer

Pages 22–23 explain how to manipulate your fiber intake according to which group you fall into. To help you achieve the fiber levels that are right for you, the recipes in this book are categorized as low, medium, or high fiber and are defined as follows:

LOW	0–3g fiber per meal
MEDIUM	3–5g fiber per meal
HIGH	5–8g fiber per meal

These will help you to reach your low, medium, or high fiber targets per day as shown above. You will also need to account for accompaniments and snacks.

You can move between low, medium, and high levels of fiber as needed by referring to the nutritional breakdown of each recipe. You can also adapt recipes to higher or lower levels of fiber by serving them with different accompaniments or omitting certain ingredients; see the tips in the recipe introductions. The recipes in the Meat and Fish chapters are mostly classed as low fiber, because meat and fish are in themselves not fibrous, but you can make these meals higher in fiber by serving with wholewheat bread, brown rice noodles, potatoes, or other vegetable or fruit accompaniments. Choose appropriately by referring to their labels and the fiber table on pages 24–25.

The sample menu planners on pages 42–43 give you an idea of how you might plan your meals according to whether you are following a low residue diet or low, medium, or high fiber diet.

You will soon become familiar with the fiber content of different foods and once you become adept at reading food labels, choosing foods with the right level of fiber for you will become second nature.

Always remember to approach the management of your IBS from a holistic perspective encompassing all the lifestyle factors as well as dietary factors dealt with in this book. Most of all remember to enjoy your food!

Sample Menus

	DAY 1	DAY 2	DAY 3
Breakfast	Toasted rice cereal (e.g. Rice Krispies) with 2% milk Fresh fruit juice	White toast with olive-oil based margarine and honey Yogurt and stewed apples	Boiled egg, broiled tomato and white toast Fresh fruit juice
Lunch	Asparagus and Potato Fritatta (page 74) White bread roll Baked apple (no skin) with honey and low-fat crème fraîche	Wild Mushroom and Tomato Soup (page 61) White crispbreads with a little cheese Fresh fruit juice	Sandwich with roasted vegetables and lean ham, made with crusty white farmhouse bread Puréed berry fruit coulis and yogurt
Dinner	Garam Masala Duck Breast (page 98) Boiled peeled potatoes Steamed vegetables Almond and Polenta Cookies (page 137) with stewed fruit (not fresh)	Baked Fish Parcel (page 88) Savory rice Stir-fried Asparagus with Sesame Seeds (page 108) Peach and Grappa Sorbet (page 134)	Asian Steamed Tofu with Mushrooms and Greens (page 112) Cherry tomatoes Steamed noodles Canned peaches and yogurt with honey

LOW FIBER (12g/½ oz. per day)

	DAY 1	DAY 2	DAY 3
Breakfast 4g	Beef and Potato Hash (page 48) Poached egg Sliced nectarine with skin	Shredded Wheat with 2% milk Apple	Healthy Eggs Florentine with wholewheat bread (page 51) Banana
Lunch 4g	Grilled sea bass or other white fish Tabbouleh (page 65) Fruit salad	Brown bread sandwich with smoked salmon and salad Grated apple (with skin) and yogurt	Wild Mushroom and Bread Salad (page 66) Wild arugula salad Grapes
Dinner 4g	Meatballs with Chickpeas (page 101) Warm white pita bread Raspberries and crème fraîche	Broiled Swordfish with Cannellini Bean Salad (page 92) White rice, green salad Strawberry Cheesecake (page 134)	Mediterranean Chicken and Prune Stew (page 104) Wholesome Mashed Tatties in their Skins (page 118) Steamed zucchini and leeks Almond and Polenta Cookies (page 137) with icecream (not fresh fruit)

MEDIUM FIBER (18g/¾oz. per day)

	DAY 1	DAY 2	DAY 3
Breakfast 6g	Apricot Muffin (page 52) Fresh fruit salad with nuts and yogurt	Kedgeree (page 51) ½ grapefruit	Wheat crackers (e.g., Wheat Thins) with 2% milk Fruit juice
Lunch 6g	Bruschetta with Chard, Borlotti Beans, and Anchovy Sauce (page 78) Apple	Warm Potato Salad with Green Beans, Scallions, and Chives (see page 67) Broiled chicken breast Fresh orange	Shrimp on Toast (see page 79) Fresh fruit salad
Dinner 6g	Persian Chicken with Rice (page 100) Green salad Strawberry Cheesecake (page 134)	Thai Noodles with Tofu and Vegetables (page 112) Tofu-sesame Dipping Sauce with Steamed Vegetables (page 117) Grapes	Broiled Swordfish with Cannellini Bean Salad (page 92) New potatoes Stir-fried Asparagus with Sesame Seeds (page 108) Peach and Grappa Sorbet (page 134)

HIGH FIBER (24g/1oz. per day)

	DAY 1	DAY 2	DAY 3
Breakfast 8g	Granola (page 54) with 2% milk	Fruit Compote (page 54) with yogurt and a little All-Bran	Wholewheat toast with poached egg, broiled bacon and tomato Melon
Lunch 8g	Rye bread with walnuts, prunes, ricotta and roasted peppers Nectarine	Tuna Niçoise with a Pulse (page 94) Banana	Potato Galette with Wholewheat Pastry (page 81) Green salad Fresh fruit salad
Dinner 8g	Broiled Polenta with Shrimp, Venetian Style (page 95) Black currant Fool (page 138)	Broiled Trout with Almonds (page 84) Couscous Broiled Eggplant with Miso (page 116) Chocolate Fridge Cake (page 137)	Middle Eastern Lamb Wrapped in Cabbage Leaves (page 103) Green leafy salad Date-filled Sticky Toffee Pudding (page 140)

I have written several healthy cookbooks and have realized how much it has affected the way I shop and cook for my family. When I worked in restaurants I would rarely cook at home. On the few occasions when I would dust off my saucepans and entertain, my menus were often elaborate and full of rich ingredients. Until I started to think about healthy food, I would often pop a carton of cream in my shopping cart and wouldn't bat an eyelid about pouring copious amounts of olive oil on any dish I was serving. Now I think differently and have felt a great deal better for it.

What I hope to have achieved with this book is to provide you with a variety of recipes to cook at home. Some are elaborate and could be used for entertaining; others are simple ideas for everyday cooking. With a family of my own I know the importance of cooking healthy, but easy dishes that everyone can enjoy. These recipes are not meant to be dull and uninspiring. I wanted to show the reader that stylish and interesting recipes could also be healthy.

While researching for this book I would often receive lots of chuckles and winks when explaining which book I was working on. I live in Wimbledon and would joke that the title could have been "Windless from Wimbledon." IBS is not something many people feel comfortable about discussing. But I was amazed by how many people were interested in the book for themselves or friends and family who suffered from it. In fact, my husband was more than happy to eat the recipes I tested and could verify the effectiveness of them. He looks forward to the sequel!

The other crucial point to make about this book is how much our diet affects this illness. A recipe book is therefore essential to help any person with IBS. This book will give you information and regimes to help keep this ailment at bay, so you can live more of a normal life.

During my research and discussions with Erica, I soon realized there was a disparity between what people perceived they could eat if they suffered from IBS and what was beneficial to them. The list of foods that people wrote down that helped and hindered was often littered with similar food items. But once Erica had explained the complexity of this illness it became apparent that there are no straightforward symptoms. It can vary from day to day; one minute you are constipated, the next minute the opposite.

So the book needed recipes that offered different levels of fiber, depending on what state your bowels were in. Hence the recipes in this book have a low-, medium- or high-fiber rating. This way you can pick and choose which recipes work for your ailments at any given time. I have then, as much as possible, given suggestions for adapting each recipe, so that you can change from low to medium to high accordingly, thus increasing the number of recipes you can use.

The next point I learned was that in order to make an effective recovery you could not do it in a hurry. You have to slowly adapt your bowels to a healthy rhythm and it's the maintenance of a healthy rhythm that is important. You could almost describe IBS as a freestyle jazz piece as opposed to a gentle Mozart concerto (no offenses to jazz intended!). But a top-performing digestive system needs to be trained and many IBS sufferers have a badly behaved delinquent inside them, not a controlled disciplined athlete. This book will help you tame the beast inside!

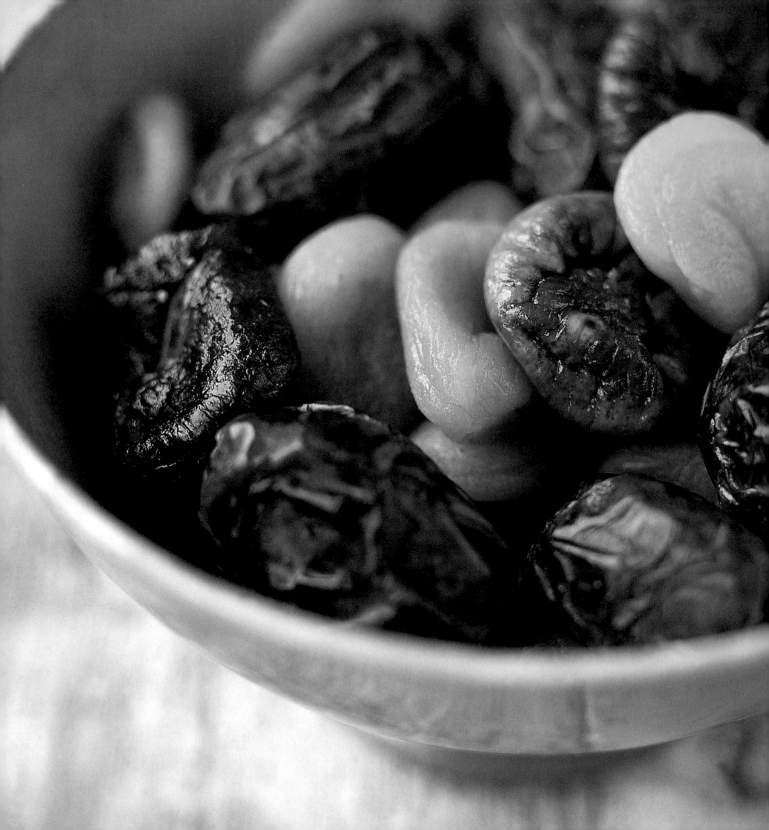

1 Breakfasts and Breads

Beef and potato hash

This dish incorporates the Pot-roasted Beef Brisket recipe on page 100, so if you have some left over use it in this recipe to make a delicious breakfast or brunch. Lovely and satisfying, especially on cold winter mornings, or as a weekend treat. **Serves 6**

14–18oz. pot-roasted beef brisket (see page 100)
6–7 medium potatoes (waxy or baking depending on how fluffy you like your hash)
8 tablespoons sunflower oil
1 large red onion, coarsely chopped
Salt and freshly ground black pepper
1 large yellow bell pepper, seeded and cut into cubes
1 large ripe tomato or 8 cherry tomatoes
Chopped flat-leaf parsley (optional)

Cook the Pot-roasted Beef Brisket according to the recipe on page 100. Remove the meat from the liquid and leave to cool, then flake 14–18oz. into chunks (you can use the rest of the meat another day).

To make the beef hash, cook the potatoes whole in their skins in boiling water with a good pinch of salt for about 20–45 minutes, depending on their size. They should be undercooked rather than overcooked. Cut into large chunks.

In a large skillet, heat the oil and fry the onion and potatoes until the potatoes are light golden brown, seasoning with salt and pepper. Reduce the heat a little, add the yellow pepper, and cook for another 5 minutes. Then add the tomato(es) and cook until any liquid has been reduced and the pepper is soft. Add the flaked beef and cook over a gentle heat for a further 5–10 minutes to allow the flavors to infuse.

Serve with chopped parsley to add color, if you wish.

Fiber rating: LOW
Per serving: 2.2g fiber, 350 Calories, 21g fat, 4g saturated fat, 0.55g sodium

Focaccia with potatoes, cherry tomatoes, and rosemary

An Italian flatbread which can also be flavored with chopped herbs, caramelized onions, or olives. Sprinkle them into the dimples or fold them into the dough just before baking. **Makes 1 x 3½-lb. loaf**

8 cups wholewheat flour
Coarse sea salt and freshly ground black pepper
1 sachet easy active dried yeast
1 teaspoon sugar
2¾ cups lukewarm water
2 tablespoons extra virgin olive oil, plus a bit extra
32–34 cherry tomatoes
1 medium cooked unpeeled potato
Several rosemary sprigs

Put the flour, 2 teaspoons salt, the yeast, sugar, water, and 1 tablespoon of the olive oil in a bowl or food processor. Knead for about 5 minutes into a soft and slightly sticky ball. Using your hand, smear a film of oil on top, to stop the dough from drying out. Cover with a dish towel and allow to rise in a warm place for about 2 hours or until doubled in size.

While the bread is rising, preheat the oven to 375°F. Put the tomatoes in a gratin dish with the remaining olive oil, salt and pepper and bake in the oven about 1–1½ hours until all the juices have evaporated and the tomatoes are caramelized. Turn the heat down if the tomatoes are starting to burn.

When the dough has risen, coarsely break up the potatoes into small pieces and fold into the dough. Lightly grease a baking sheet with olive oil and spread the dough out to form a round of about 12–18 inches diameter. Dot over the tomatoes, smashing them into the bread, and smear any cooking juices from them over the top: this is the tastiest bit. Scatter over the rosemary sprigs and finally season with salt and pepper. **Increase** the oven temperature to 400°F. Leave the dough to rise again for about 30 minutes. Once it has risen a second time, bake in the oven for about 20 minutes, or until golden brown. As soon as it comes out of the oven, drizzle a little olive oil over it and leave to cool for 10 minutes before serving warm.

Fiber rating: LOW
Per 35g slice: 2.2g fiber, 81 Calories, 1g fat, 0g saturated fat, 0.08g sodium

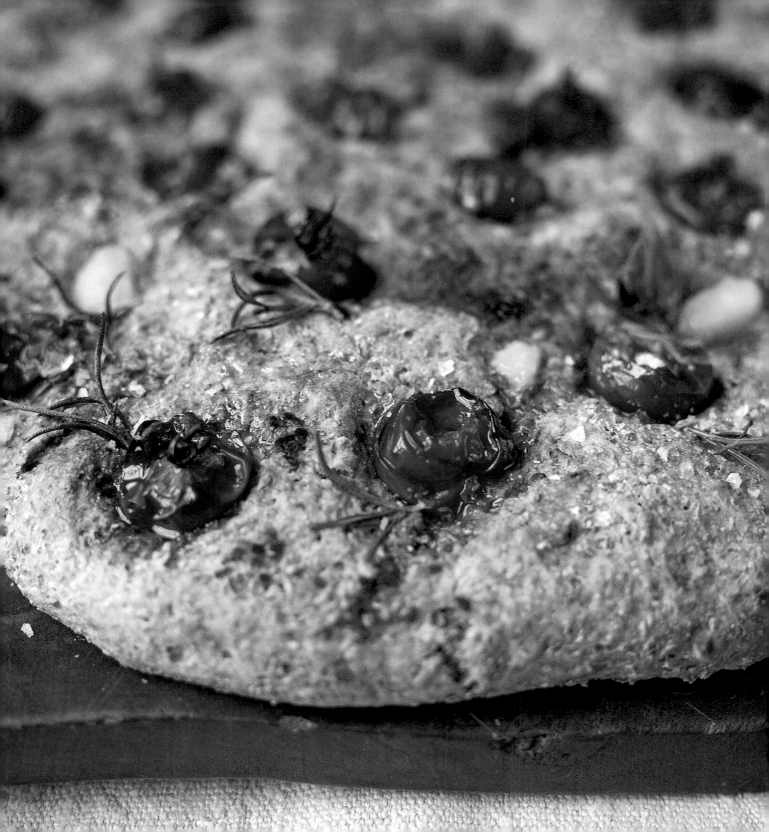

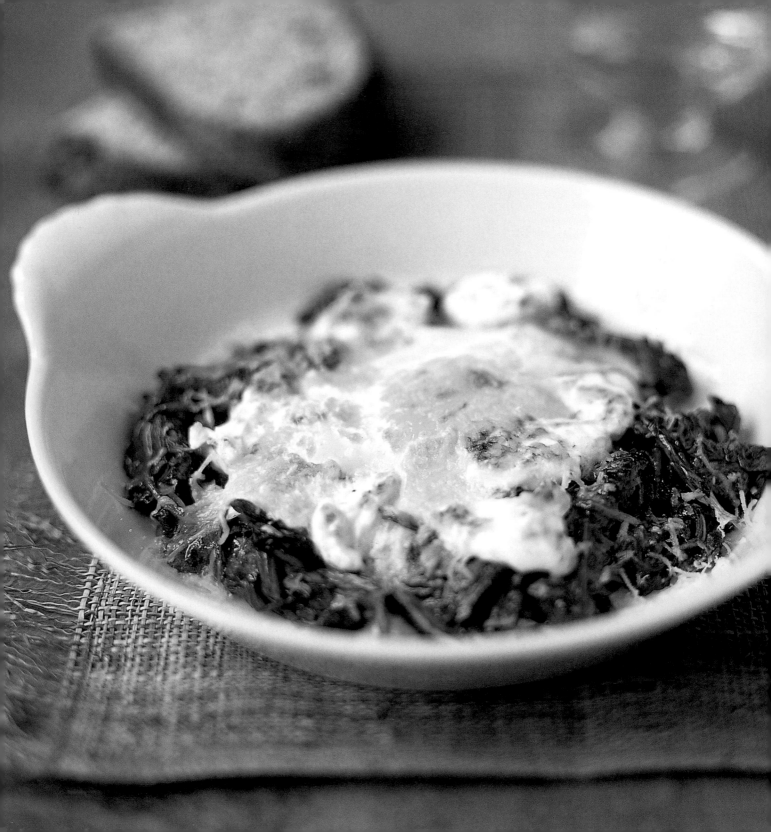

Healthy eggs florentine

This is a simple and healthy version of an egg dish often found on traditional Italian menus in England. It may be cooked in small individual dishes or one larger gratin dish about 8–10 inches across. Alternatively you could use small or medium oven-proof skillets. **Serves 4**

5–6 cups spinach, washed and drained
Salt and freshly ground black pepper
½ cup ricotta cheese
8 large basil leaves, finely chopped (optional)
4 eggs
5 tablespoons grated Parmesan
4 medium slices warm crusty brown bread

Don't bother to trim the spinach stems unless they are very large and tough. Tear the leaves a bit if they are large, or just buy small-leafed spinach for ease.

In a large saucepan or skillet, cook the spinach in batches, stirring frequently until it is wilted. Spinach has enough moisture in it not to need extra water. Place in a colander until all the spinach is cooked, then squeeze dry, pressing out any excess water.

Preheat the grill to high. Place the warm spinach leaves in four individual heatproof dishes or one large gratin dish and season with salt and pepper.

Put the ricotta in a bowl and mix with the chopped basil leaves, if using, and season with salt and pepper.

Carefully break the eggs over the spinach without breaking the yolks and dollop the ricotta around the sides with a little on top of the yolks. Scatter over the Parmesan and place under the grill. Cook for 2–4 minutes until the eggs are just set but still soft in the middle.

Serve right away with the warm bread.

Fiber rating: MEDIUM
Per serving including bread: 4.8g fiber, 262 Calories, 13g fat, 5g saturated fat, 1.02g sodium

Kedgeree

In this version of the Anglo-Indian classic, brown or white basmati rice can be used and the lentils omitted, depending on your fiber needs. The trick to cooking brown rice successfully is to use just enough water. It becomes waterlogged very easily and loses its nutty, light appeal. **Serves 4**

¾ cup brown basmati rice
½ cup green or Puy lentils
Pinch of turmeric (optional)
1 medium onion, finely chopped
1 teaspoon ground cumin
1 teaspoon ground coriander
3 tablespoons sunflower oil or ½ stick unsalted butter
11oz. smoked haddock fillet, skinned, and thickly sliced
2 eggs (optional)
½ oz. fresh cilantro, roughly chopped

Place the rice and lentils in a saucepan and add about 2 cups hot water. Add the turmeric, if using, and give the rice and lentils a good stir. Cover with a lid and bring to a boil, then gently simmer for about 20–25 minutes until the rice is just cooked and the lentils are soft. Remove from the heat and leave with the lid on to steam for 10 minutes. If there is still water left in the pan, cook gently until it has all evaporated.

Cook the onion, cumin, and ground coriander in the oil or butter in a large high-sided skillet or saucepan for about 10 minutes, until soft and translucent. Increase the heat to high, add the haddock and cook for a few minutes. When the haddock is just cooked, push to the side and break the eggs, if using, into the saucepan. Cook the eggs until the whites start to turn solid. Break the yolks to help them cook more quickly. When the eggs are just cooked, briefly stir into the haddock mixture, trying to leave large pieces of egg.

Add the rice and lentils to the haddock mixture with half the chopped cilantro. Mix briefly until just incorporated. Return to the heat if not hot enough.

Serve with the remaining chopped cilantro, wedges of lemon, buttered toast, and relish.

Fiber rating: MEDIUM
Per serving including eggs, not including serving suggestion: 3g fiber, 414 Calories, 17g fat, 5g saturated fat, 0.61g sodium

Wholewheat soda bread with seeds and grains

Soda bread is quick and easy to make. This version is delicious served with smoked salmon for a decadent breakfast or brunch. It also makes great toast.

Makes 1 x 1¾-lb. loaf

3½ cups wholewheat flour or granary flour
1 cup bran
1 cup barley flakes (optional)
⅔ cup sunflower or pumpkin seeds (reserve 1 tablespoon for topping if you wish)
2 heaping teaspoons sea salt
1 heaping teaspoon baking powder
1 heaping teaspoon sodium bicarbonate or baking soda
Scant ¾ cup low-fat plain yogurt
¾ cup warm water
Oil, for greasing

Preheat the oven to 375°F. Lightly oil a large flat roasting sheet and place in the oven.

Place the dry ingredients in a large bowl or in a food processor with a dough hook. Mix briefly, then add the yogurt and water. Mix until well incorporated and knead for a few minutes.

When a firm but slightly sticky lump of dough has formed, shape it into a ball. Scatter over the reserved seeds, if using, or dust with flour. Place on the preheated sheet and bake for about 40 minutes, until golden brown. Tap the base to check that it sounds hollow and is cooked through.

Transfer to a wire rack and allow to cool for at least 30 minutes before slicing and eating.

Fiber rating: MEDIUM
Per 40g slice: 3.4g fiber, 110 Calories, 3g fat, 0g saturated fat, 0.3g sodium

Apricot muffins

A tasty breakfast or snack. Other dried fruit can be substituted for the apricots, as well as other fresh fruit such as bananas or papaya. The bran included increases the insoluble fiber content. For a low fiber version use all-purpose flour instead of wholewheat flour. **Makes 10–12 medium muffins**

5 tablespoons sunflower oil, plus extra for greasing
2 medium eggs
¾ cup superfine sugar
⅔ cup low-fat plain yogurt
1 heaping cup wholewheat or all-purpose flour, sifted
1 cup bran
1 heaping teaspoon baking powder
Pinch of baking soda (optional)
½ cup dried apricots, chopped
Pinch of ground ginger and/or cinnamon
2 tablespoons chopped roasted nuts, such as almonds or hazelnuts

Preheat the oven to 375°F. Grease 12 muffin molds with sunflower oil.

Whisk the eggs and sugar together until they double in volume or form a ribbon consistency.

Add the sunflower oil, yogurt, sifted flour, bran, baking powder, baking soda, if using, chopped apricots, ginger and/or cinnamon, and half the nuts. Fold the mixture gently until just incorporated (do not beat) and spoon into the muffin molds, so that it is just level with the top. Scatter over the remaining nuts.

Bake in the oven for about 15 minutes until the mixture is just firm and golden brown. Allow to rest in the molds for 5 minutes. Then turn out on to a wire rack to cool, or eat right away.

Fiber rating: MEDIUM
Per muffin, with wholewheat flour: 3.9g fiber, 241 Calories, 11g fat, 2g saturated fat, 0.12g sodium

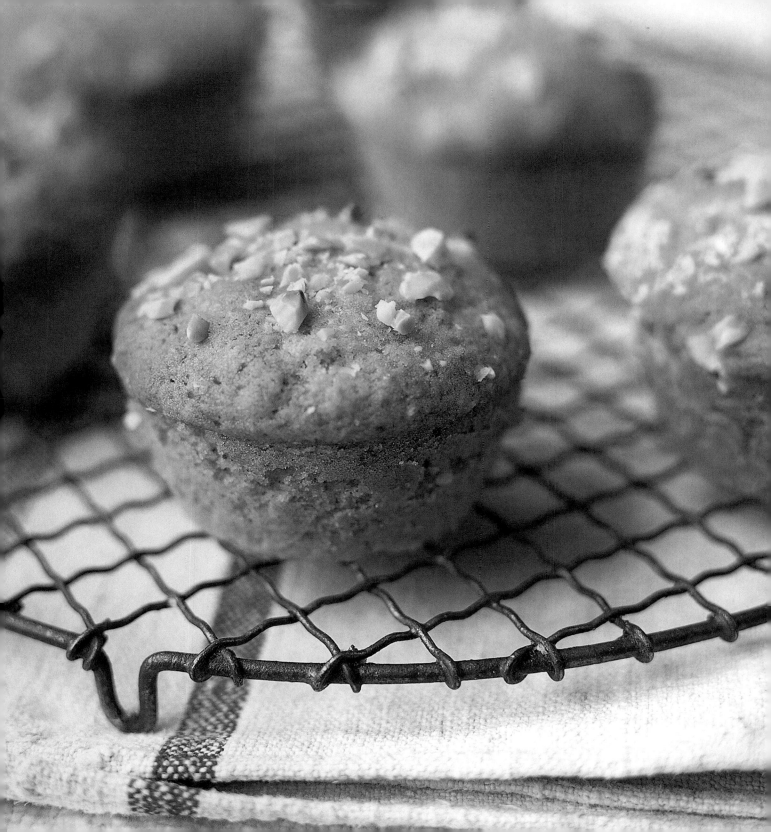

Granola

There are many good varieties of granola on the market, but most are high in soluble fiber. This one is high in insoluble fiber. Play around with ingredients to suit you; try experimenting with other grains such as quinoa. The ingredients can easily be increased if you need to make a big batch. **Serves 4**

1 cup bran flakes

⅓ cup rolled oats

⅓ cup roasted coconut flakes

⅓ cup wheat germ

⅓ cup dried chopped apricots

¼ cup brown rice flakes

¼ cup unskinned roasted almonds, coarsely chopped

Mix all the ingredients together and store in an airtight container to keep fresh.

Serve with just milk or yogurt, or even Fruit Compote (see right), depending on your fiber requirements.

Fiber rating: HIGH

Per serving: 5g fiber, 195 Calories, 7g fat, 2g saturated fat, 0.11g sodium

Fruit compote

A simple dish to prepare in advance and keep in the fridge for at least two weeks. Serve for breakfast with yogurt as well as some good-quality granola (see left) that includes nuts. It's also delicious as a healthy dessert.

Serves 4

½ cup dried pineapple

½ cup dried apricots, quartered

½ cup dried peaches or mango, quartered

½ cup dried cherries or cranberries

¼ cup raisins

1 cup apple juice or water

1 small cinnamon stick

½ vanilla bean

2 pieces preserved ginger, finely chopped

For serving

¾ cup low-fat plain yogurt

Good-quality granola (optional—see left)

⅓ cup blanched almonds, coarsely chopped and roasted in a medium oven for 10 minutes

Place the dried fruits in a saucepan and add the apple juice or water, cinnamon, and vanilla. Bring to a boil, then simmer gently for 10 minutes. Add the ginger off the heat and leave to cool.

Store in an airtight container in the fridge and use as needed.

Serve a large spoonful on top of some yogurt or good-quality granola and chopped nuts for a nourishing breakfast.

Fiber rating: HIGH

Per serving, not including granola: 6g fiber, 278 Calories, 8g fat, 1g saturated fat, 0.05g sodium

Chickpea flat bread

The Indians use a lot of chickpea (or gram) flour and these are moreish little pancakes to serve with any Indian-style dish or just with a dollop of yogurt and good-quality relish for a snack. You can buy chickpea flour in health food and Asian food stores. **Serves 4**

2 cups chickpea flour
2 garlic cloves, finely chopped
1 teaspoon finely grated fresh
   ginger root (optional)
2 heaping tablespoons
   coarsely chopped cilantro
½ cup low-fat plain yogurt

Large pinch of salt
Sunflower oil, for frying
For serving (optional)
Yogurt, diced tomatoes, thinly
   sliced scallions or red
   onions, cilantro sprigs and
   lime relish

Place the chickpea flour in a bowl and add the garlic, ginger, if using, cilantro, yogurt, and salt. Pour in 1 cup of the water and slowly mix together to form a thick batter without lumps. Add more water if too thick.

Heat a skillet and lightly grease with sunflower oil. Pour in the chickpea batter, about 1 tablespoon at a time, to form small thin pancakes. Cook the pancakes for 3 minutes on each side until lightly browned. As you cook, set the pancakes aside on a warm plate until you have used up all the batter.

Serve the pancakes with yogurt, tomatoes, onions, cilantro sprigs, and relish on top.

Fiber rating: HIGH
Per serving, not including serving suggestion: 6.8g fiber, 216 Calories, 4g fat, 1g saturated fat, 0.33g sodium

Rye bread with figs and walnuts

Like all wheat-free breads, this can seem a little on the heavy side, so substitute half the rye flour with granary flour if you prefer (this will give you similar levels of fiber). Other dried fruit can be used instead of figs if you wish. **Makes 1 x 1½-lb. loaf**

5 cups rye flour
2 cups walnut pieces
⅔ cup dried figs, coarsely
   chopped
2 teaspoons dried yeast

1 heaping teaspoon sea salt
1 teaspoon brown sugar
1¼ cups warm water
Oil, for greasing

Place the dry ingredients in a large bowl, or in a food processor with a dough hook, and mix briefly. Add the water and gently mix into a firm sticky dough that holds its shape.

Place the dough on a lightly greased baking sheet, forming a round bread shape. Make a cross on the top with a knife and sprinkle with a little flour. Allow to rise, or increase a little in size, in a warm place for about 1–2 hours.

Preheat the oven to 375°F.

Bake the bread in the oven for about 30–45 minutes. Remove from the oven and tap the base to check that it sounds hollow and is cooked.

Transfer to a wire rack and leave to cool for at least 30 minutes before slicing and eating. This bread is also delicious toasted.

Fiber rating: HIGH
Per 2 x 1 oz. slice: 6.9g fiber, 247 Calories, 6g fat, 1g saturated fat, 0.2g sodium

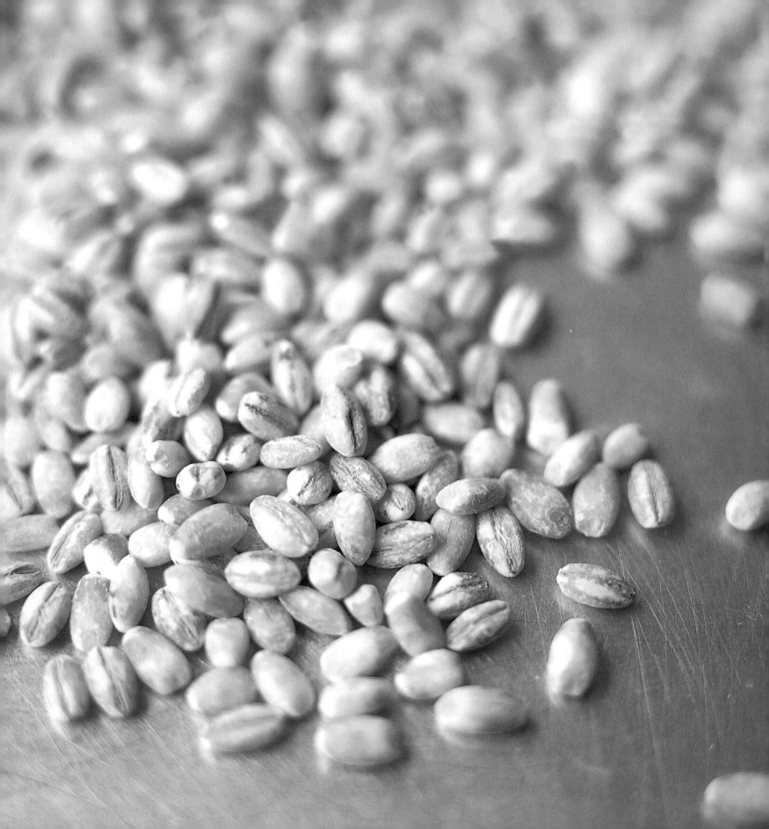

Soups and Salads

2

Minestrone with barley

Italians use pasta, rice, pulses, or bread in their minestrone to make it a meal in itself. But you can substitute any pulse, e.g. cannellini or borlotti beans, if you want to increase your fiber intake. Try chard as a change from broccoli if you prefer the look. **Serves 6**

4 tablespoons extra virgin olive oil	1 small head broccoli, divided into small florets
½ cup smoked streaky bacon, diced	2 garlic cloves, chopped
1 large red onion, finely chopped	Salt and freshly ground black pepper
2 medium carrots, finely chopped (unpeeled)	½ cup barley
2 celery sticks, finely chopped	1 tablespoon chopped thyme
2 cups green beans, finely chopped	4 cups chicken stock or water
2 large zucchini, finely chopped	Drizzle of extra virgin olive oil or fresh pesto sauce, to serve (optional)

In a heavy saucepan, heat the olive oil over a medium heat and cook the bacon, briefly. Add the onion, followed by the rest of the vegetables, adding each after you have chopped them, starting with the carrots and finishing with the garlic. Stir briefly after each addition. Once all the vegetables are added, season with salt and pepper and cook gently for 10 minutes, stirring occasionally.

Add the barley and thyme, mix and cook a further few minutes to coat the barley in oil.

Add the chicken stock or water and simmer gently for about 40 minutes, until all the vegetables are tender and the barley is soft.

Serve the soup with a drizzle of extra virgin olive oil or pesto sauce if you like. This soup tastes even better if prepared in advance, giving the flavors a chance to develop.

Fiber rating: MEDIUM
Per serving: 3.9g fiber, 138 Calories, 10g fat, 2g saturated fat, 0.75g sodium

Soba noodle broth with chicken

Use any noodles to suit your tastes or fiber needs. Wholewheat or faro noodles would increase the fiber; buckwheat soba noodles and rice noodles are good options if you are trying to avoid wheat. Beef fillet can replace the chicken if you prefer. **Serves 4**

3 cups buckwheat soba noodles	2 scallions, sliced at an angle
2 medium chicken breasts (9oz.)	1 handful sugar snap peas, halved or 2 handfuls baby spinach leaves
Dash of oil, for cooking	1 teaspoon hoisin sauce
2½ cups chicken stock	4 tablespoons mirin or sherry
12 shiitake mushrooms, quartered or halved depending on size	4 tablespoons Japanese dark soy sauce
	Few cilantro sprigs

Cook the noodles in lots of lightly salted water following the manufacturer's instructions; take care not to overcook. Drain, refresh in cold water and place in a bowl. Soba noodles can easily stick together like glue, so handle them carefully and leave some water in the bowl to keep them moist.

Heat a griddle until hot and smear the chicken with a little oil to prevent it sticking. Broil the chicken for about 5 minutes each side or until cooked through. Set aside to rest and slice just before serving.

Have all the prepared vegetables to hand before you start to cook them as they are cooked very quickly.

Bring the stock to a boil and add the mushrooms, hoisin sauce, mirin, and soy sauce.

While the stock is coming to a boil again, refresh the noodles in hot or boiling water, drain well and divide among four warmed soup bowls. When the stock boils, quickly add the scallions and peas or spinach. Remove the stock from the heat and, with a slotted spoon, divide the vegetables between the soup bowls. Scatter over the sliced chicken and finally pour over the stock. Garnish with a few sprigs of cilantro and serve.

Fiber rating: LOW
Per serving: 1.8g fiber, 358 Calories, 3g fat, 1g saturated fat, 0.72g sodium

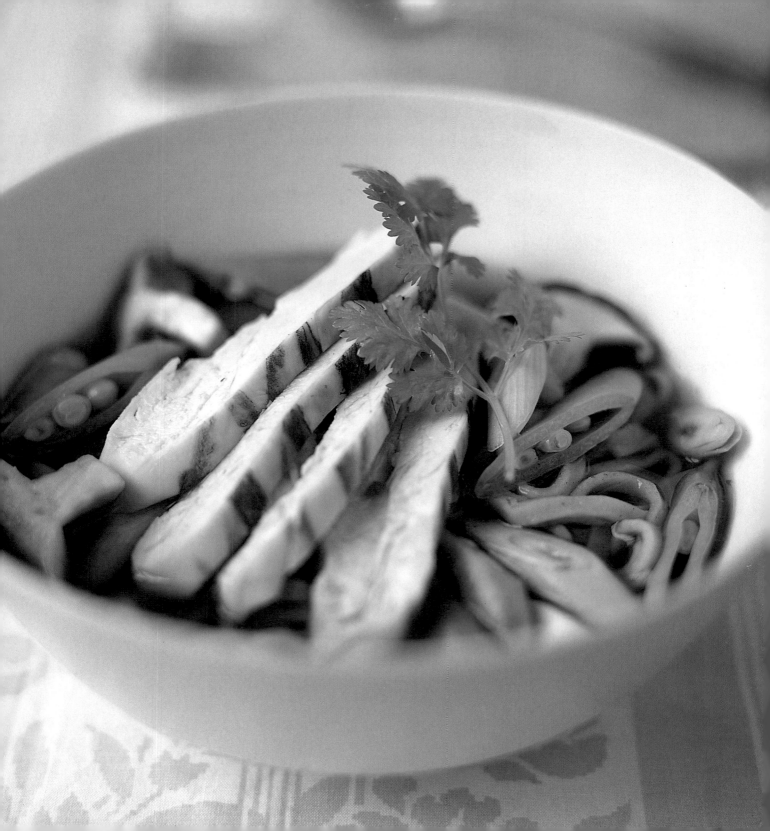

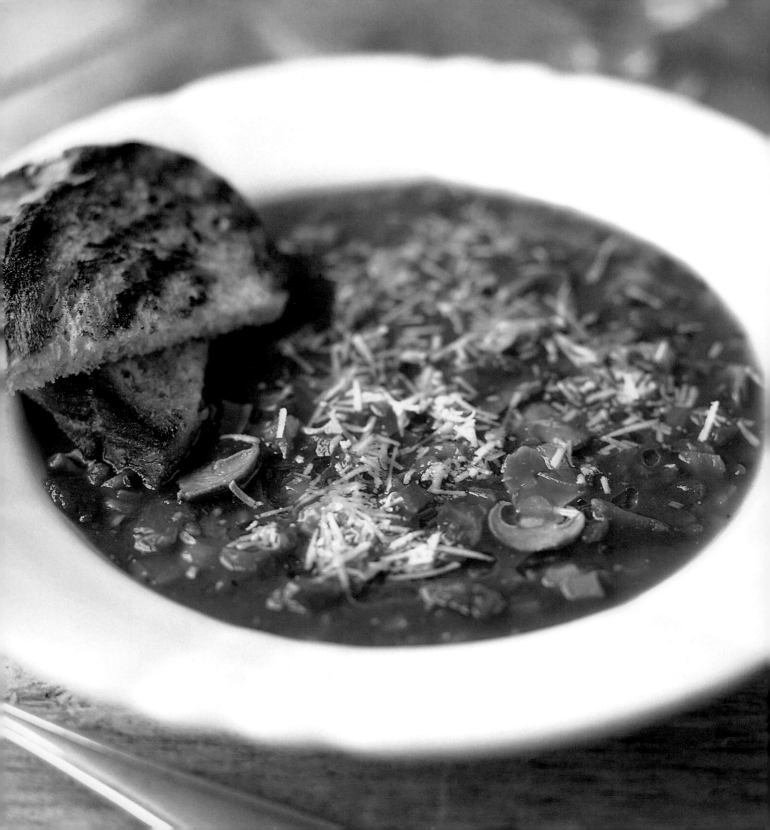

Wild mushroom and tomato soup

Mushrooms are a low-fiber vegetable so the fiber in this recipe comes from the bread. It is a traditional Italian soup using dried mushrooms which have a more robust flavor than ordinary mushrooms. Use Italian dried porcini for best results. **Serves 4**

4 tablespoons extra virgin olive oil

1 large red onion, finely chopped

3 celery sticks, finely chopped

2 garlic cloves, finely chopped

3 rosemary sprigs, finely chopped

Salt and freshly ground black pepper

Generous 1oz. dried porcini mushrooms, soaked for 15 minutes in just enough hot water to cover

²/₃ cup red or white wine

14-oz. can tomatoes or fresh tomatoes, peeled and cubed

To serve

4 slices sourdough bread (optional)

1 garlic clove, halved (optional)

¹/₃ cup Parmesan cheese, grated

Drizzle of extra virgin olive oil

Heat the olive oil in a saucepan and add the chopped onion and celery. Cook at a gentle simmer for about 15 minutes until they are soft and translucent. Add the garlic and rosemary and cook a minute more. Season with salt and pepper.

Drain the porcini, reserving the soaking liquid, and add to the saucepan, mixing for a few minutes. Add the soaking liquid, discarding any sediment, and pour in the wine. Bring to a boil and cook gently until the liquid has reduced back into the mushrooms.

Add the tomatoes to the pan and simmer gently until they are reduced to a thick sauce. Then add about 2 cups of water and simmer gently for another 20 minutes.

Toast the bread and rub with the cut side of the halved garlic clove while still warm. Pour the soup into serving bowls, scatter with Parmesan, drizzle a little extra virgin olive oil on top if you like, and serve with the bread.

Fiber rating: MEDIUM

Per serving including bread: 3.9g fiber, 343 Calories, 14g fat, 4g saturated fat, 0.59g sodium

Watercress and fennel soup with Indian spices

Many lettuces have no nutritional or fiber value. Watercress is one of the few exceptions. The potatoes are unpeeled to increase the fiber content and make the recipe easier. **Serves 2**

2 tablespoons extra virgin olive or sunflower oil

1 medium onion, chopped

1 medium bulb fennel, chopped

2 small potatoes (3½ oz.)

2 small garlic cloves, chopped

3 cups chicken stock or water

2 medium bunches watercress

To serve (optional)

2 heaping tablespoons low-fat plain live yogurt

½ teaspoon garam masala (see page 98)

1 tablespoon chopped fennel fonds or dill

Heat the oil in a medium saucepan and gently cook the onion, fennel, potatoes, and garlic covered with a lid for about 15 minutes until the vegetables are transparent and nearly cooked. Stir periodically to prevent them from burning. Add the stock or water, bring to a boil and simmer for about 10 minutes until the potatoes are soft.

Wash and roughly chop the watercress. Add to the pan of vegetables and cook for 5 minutes. Turn off the heat and blend until completely puréed for best results. Using a food processor will not purée the watercress completely.

Serve hot or at room temperature, but do not reheat for long or the vibrant color will deteriorate.

Top the soup with a dollop of yogurt mixed with garam masala, if you wish, and chopped fennel fronds or dill.

Fiber rating: MEDIUM

Per serving not including serving suggestion: 4.8g fiber, 200 Calories, 13g fat, 2g saturated fat, 0.71g sodium

Chilled beet and dill soup
Beets are cleansing vegetables and make a comforting soup, which can be served either hot or cold. Any kind of stock can be used instead of chicken, including vegetable stock if you are looking for a vegetarian option. **Serves 4**

1 large red onion, finely chopped
2 garlic cloves, chopped
3 tablespoons olive oil
3 cups beets, cooked in water, not in vinegar
Salt and freshly ground black pepper

3½ cups light chicken stock
1 heaping teaspoon cornstarch (if serving the soup hot)
¾ cup low-fat plain set yogurt
1 heaping tablespoon chopped dill or mint

Gently cook the onion and garlic in the olive oil until the onion is soft and transparent.

Peel the beet, cut off the ends and wash. Chop the beetroot into small pieces, add to the onion and cook gently for 5 minutes. Season with salt and pepper.

Add the chicken stock and bring to a boil. Simmer for about 10 minutes to infuse the flavor of the beets. Set aside.

Purée the soup in batches in a food processor or in a blender for finer results. Add a little more water if necessary, though this soup is best served thick. Taste and adjust the seasoning as required.

If serving the soup hot, stir the tablespoon of cornstarch into ⅔ cup of the yogurt. Add this yogurt to the last batch of soup being liquidized. Pour the soup back into the saucepan and cook gently for 2 minutes to reheat and cook the cornstarch. **If** serving the soup cold, make sure it has cooled before adding ⅔ cup of the yogurt to the last batch of soup before blending.

Serve warm or chilled with a dollop of yogurt and some chopped dill or mint on top.

Fiber rating: MEDIUM
Per serving: 4.2g fiber, 218 Calories, 10g fat, 2g saturated fat, 0.99g sodium

Tomato and tamarind soup
Tamarind is used in Asian cooking and can be found in Oriental shops and some supermarkets. It has a distinct sour flavor, which works well with sweet tomatoes. Tamarind paste, as opposed to whole tamarind, is the easiest way of using this spice. **Serves 4**

½ cup green Puy lentils
4 tablespoons sunflower or olive oil
2 garlic cloves
1 medium onion, finely chopped
2 teaspoons ground cumin seeds, toasted
1 teaspoon mustard seeds

4 cups canned tomatoes
1 heaping tablespoon tamarind paste
1 large chile, finely chopped (optional)
For serving (optional)
Coarsely chopped cilantro
Low-fat plain live yogurt
Naan or flatbread

First cook the lentils in a saucepan of water until tender. Do not add salt or they will take ages to cook, but season the water with a dash of oil and 1 of the garlic cloves to add flavor and help soften the lentil skins.

Heat the oil in another saucepan and gently cook the onion for about 10 minutes until soft. Add the remaining garlic, the cumin and mustard seeds and cook for a few more minutes.

Add the tomatoes to the spicy onion and cook for about 15 minutes, to reduce the liquid and intensify the flavor, making a sweet sauce.

Add the tamarind paste, cooked lentils and chile, if using. Cook the mixture for about 5 minutes, then add about 2 cups of water. Season with salt and pepper if liked and cook for about 15 minutes to infuse the flavors. Add more water if need be, though this is a soup that should be quite thick.

Serve each bowl of soup topped with chopped cilantro, a dollop of yogurt and accompanied by naan or flatbread for a complete meal.

Fiber rating: MEDIUM
Per serving not including serving suggestion: 4.2g fiber, 230 Calories, 12g fat, 2g saturated fat, 0.09g sodium

Chicken broth with broccoli and cannellini beans

An Italian soup traditionally made with the new season's extra virgin olive oil. Omit the cannellini beans for a more authentic recipe, though they do provide extra fiber. Serves 4

- 4 heaping tablespoons cooked cannellini beans
- 4 thick slices country-style white bread
- 1 large garlic clove
- 4 cups homemade chicken stock
- Dash of sherry or vermouth
- Few slices dried wild mushrooms (optional)
- 2 cups broccoli
- Salt and freshly ground black pepper
- 1/3 cup Parmesan cheese, grated
- Drizzle of good-quality, single-estate new season's extra virgin olive oil

If using canned cannellini beans, rinse well with hot water and drain. Set aside.

Toast the bread and, while it is still hot, rub both sides with the cut side of the garlic. Cut in half and place two halves in each of four warmed shallow soup bowls. Add the cannellini beans and keep warm.

Pour the chicken stock into a saucepan, add the sherry or vermouth and the wild mushrooms, if using, and bring to a boil.

While the stock is heating, steam the broccoli for about 5 minutes. The broccoli should be cooked completely to bring out its flavor; only pasta is cooked al dente in Italy.

Place the broccoli on top of the beans and bread, season with salt and pepper, and pour over the hot stock. Sprinkle with the Parmesan, drizzle over the olive oil and serve immediately.

Fiber rating: HIGH
Per serving: 6.1g fiber, 207 Calories, 4g fat, 2g saturated fat, 0.77g sodium

Pea and tarragon soup

This soup may be served hot, at room temperature or chilled. Frozen peas are easier to deal with than fresh ones and make a greener-colored soup. Serve with wholewheat bread or croûtons to increase the fiber. Serves 4

- 3 scallions, or 1 small onion, finely chopped
- 2 tablespoons extra virgin olive oil
- 2 medium potatoes (9oz.), scrubbed well and cubed
- Salt and freshly ground black pepper
- 1 large garlic clove, chopped
- 4 cups peas
- 3½ cups chicken stock
- 4 tablespoons chopped tarragon
- 3/4 cup low-fat plain live yogurt

Cook the scallions or onion in the olive oil in a saucepan for 5 minutes on a medium-high heat. Add the cubed potatoes and garlic, season with salt and pepper and cook for 10 minutes, stirring periodically to prevent them sticking to the base of the pan.

If using fresh peas, add them to the pan and cook for a further 5 minutes. Add the chicken stock and simmer for 15 minutes. If using frozen peas, add after cooking the potatoes for 10 minutes and cook a further 5 minutes. Check that the potatoes are soft, add the tarragon and purée in a blender (not a food processor) for the best results.

Taste the soup and adjust the seasoning as necessary. If serving hot, top each bowlful with a dollop of yogurt. If serving chilled, add the yogurt to the soup once cooled and mix well. I like this soup best at room temperature.

Fiber rating: HIGH
Per serving: 6.1g fiber, 202 Calories, 7g fat, 1g saturated fat, 0.9g sodium

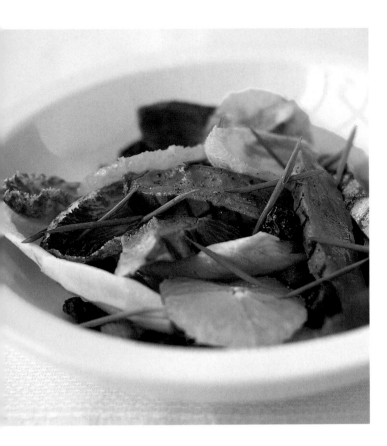

Broiled duck breast salad with endive and oranges

There is a beautiful variety of colors in this salad, particularly if you use a mixture of red and green endive. Warm Potato Salad (see page 67) makes a good accompaniment. **Serves 4 as an appetizer or 2 as main dish**

2 large duck breasts, skinless if possible

2 small oranges (blood oranges when in season look great)

½ cup blueberries or dried cherries

½ cup roasted almonds or cashew nuts

4 small to medium endive (thick-stemmed variety)

4 tablespoons extra virgin olive oil

2 tablespoons chopped chives or chervil

Salt and freshly ground black pepper

Skin the duck breasts if necessary. Heat a griddle and cook the duck on a medium-high heat for about 10 minutes, turning halfway through. I prefer my duck pink in the middle; cook a few minutes more if you want it cooked through. Set aside to rest.

Top and tail the oranges and remove the skin and pith with a serrated knife, trimming down the sides. Cut the orange in half around the equator and slice. Place in a salad bowl along with the blueberries or cherries and nuts.

Cut the endive into large pieces, or leave the leaves whole. Add to the orange salad, mix well and add the olive oil, chives or chervil, and salt and pepper. Mix briefly and transfer the salad to serving plates, leaving the dressing in the bowl.

Slice the duck and add it to the dressing, mix briefly, then scatter it over the salad. Serve right away.

Fiber rating: LOW

Per serving (appetizer): 2.7g fiber, 313 Calories, 23g fat, 4g saturated fat, 0.19g sodium

Tabbouleh
An easy salad that works well with plain grilled meat or fish or as part of a selection of mezze (Middle Eastern starters). Traditionally very little bulgur wheat is used, and plenty of fresh herbs. For a higher fiber content, use wholewheat bulgur wheat (found in good Middle Eastern stores). **Serves 4**

¼ cup bulgur wheat
Bunch (4½ oz.) flat-leaf parsley
Bunch (3½ oz.) mint
Juice of 1 large lemon

1 large tomato or 12 cherry tomatoes, finely diced
3 tablespoons extra virgin olive oil
Salt and freshly ground black pepper

Soak the bulgur wheat in just enough hot water to cover. Leave for 10 minutes and drain well, pressing out as much water as possible. Set aside.

Discard the stems of the herbs and rinse the leaves. Place on a dish towel and leave to dry thoroughly—but be careful not to bruise the leaves or they will turn brown and discolor the salad.

Once the herbs are dry, chop coarsely and place in a bowl. Add the lemon juice, diced tomatoes, olive oil, bulgur wheat, salt and pepper. Mix well and serve. The tabbouleh will keep for several hours, during which time the flavors will develop further.

Fiber rating: LOW
Per serving: 2.2g fiber, 126 Calories, 9g fat, 1g saturated fat, 0.31g sodium

Zucchini and cumin salad
Zucchini are another example of a low-fiber vegetable. For a higher fiber content, serve with warm pita bread. This salad works well with simply broiled fish or chicken, or as part of a Middle Eastern mezze meal. **Serves 4**

4 medium zucchini
Salt and freshly ground black pepper
1 tablespoon cumin seeds
1 large garlic clove, crushed with salt

¾ cup low-fat plain live yogurt
1 tablespoon extra virgin olive oil (optional)
3 heaping tablespoons coarsely chopped mint

Coarsely grate the zucchini and mix with 1 tablespoon of salt. Leave in a colander to drain for 10 minutes. This releases excess water from the zucchini.

Lightly brown the cumin seeds in a dry skillet and then grind in a spice grinder or using a pestle and mortar. Mix with the crushed garlic, yogurt, olive oil, if using, and salt and pepper.

Squeeze any remaining water from the zucchini with your hands—the salad should not be too wet. Mix the zucchini with the yogurt mixture and stir in the mint before serving.

Fiber rating: LOW
Per serving: 1.2g fiber, 77 Calories, 4g fat, 1g saturated fat, 0.23g sodium

Wild mushroom and bread salad

If fresh wild mushrooms are in season, omit dried mushrooms completely, using 18oz. mushrooms in total. I have also used leftover foccacia for this recipe (see page 48)—remove the tomatoes and add to the salad before marinating. **Serves 4**

7oz. decrusted Italian bread, e.g. ciabatta, focaccia

18oz. mushrooms, such as field, shiitake, or chestnut

2 plus 5 tablespoons extra virgin olive oil

2 large garlic cloves, finely chopped

1 heaping tablespoon chopped sage or rosemary

Salt and freshly ground black pepper

Generous 1oz. dried porcini mushrooms, soaked in just enough hot water to cover

3 tablespoons balsamic vinegar

Baby spinach or arugula leaves, for serving

Preheat the oven to 375°F. Cut or tear the bread into 1-inch cubes. Place on a baking tray and cook in the oven for about 15 minutes until golden brown and crisp on the outside.

Slice the mushrooms and cook in batches in a large skillet with 1 tablespoon of the oil: add just enough mushrooms to cover the base of the pan each time and stir frequently, frying for about 1–2 minutes. When all the mushrooms are nearly cooked, add half the garlic and half the sage or rosemary, season, cook briefly, then spoon into a large bowl.

Drain the porcini and reserve the soaking liquid. Add 1 tablespoon of the oil to the skillet and cook the porcini with the remaining garlic and sage or rosemary for a minute. Add the reserved soaking liquid and reduce back into the porcini. When the liquid has nearly disappeared, add the cooked fresh mushrooms back to the pan and mix briefly to coat in the tasty liquid. Spoon all the mushrooms back into the large bowl and add the cooked bread, balsamic vinegar, remaining 5 tablespoons olive oil, salt and pepper. Mix well and leave to marinate for at least 30 minutes before serving.

Serve the salad on the spinach or arugula leaves.

Fiber rating: LOW
Per serving: 2.2g fibre, 461 Calories, 27g fat, 4g saturated fat, 0.53g sodium

Spinach, fennel, and lentil salad

To make this fresh-tasting salad more substantial, add 1¼ cups diced, cooked bacon or 3½ cups cooked peeled shrimp. Pan-fry in a dash of olive oil and scatter over the lentils, with a squeeze of extra lemon juice. **Serves 4 as an appetizer or 2 as a main dish**

½ cup green or Puy lentils

1 garlic clove, unpeeled

5 tablespoons extra virgin olive oil

4 tablespoons lemon juice or red wine vinegar

Salt and freshly ground black pepper

1½ cups baby spinach leaves, washed

9-oz. bulb fennel

2 tablespoons coarsely chopped basil, mint or parsley

Place the lentils in a saucepan of water with the whole unpeeled garlic clove. Bring to a boil and simmer for about 30 minutes until just soft. Drain well, remove the skin from the garlic and return the lentils to the saucepan, smashing the garlic and stirring it in to flavor them. Add 2 tablespoons of the olive oil and 2 tablespoons of the lemon juice or vinegar; season with salt and pepper.

Place the spinach leaves in a large mixing bowl. Remove any green fonds from the fennel, chop them and add to the lentils. Remove the triangular heart from the fennel and thinly slice the rest of the bulb. Add to the spinach leaves and add the remaining olive oil and lemon juice or vinegar; season with salt and pepper. Mix well and place on a large plate or individual plates.

Just before serving, mix the herbs with the lentils (if you add them too far in advance they may discolor.) Scatter the lentils over the spinach and fennel salad, and serve ideally while the lentils are warm.

Fiber rating: MEDIUM
Per serving (appetizer): 4.5g fiber, 217 Calories, 15g fat, 2g saturated fat, 0.15g sodium

Warm potato salad with green beans, scallions, and chives

For best results, choose good-quality waxy potatoes that don't break up when boiled. Fresh new potatoes or salad potatoes are good examples. Serve with broiled meats or fish. **Serves 4**

18oz. waxy potatoes
Salt and freshly ground black pepper
2 cups green beans
2 scallions or 2 shallots

2 heaping tablespoons chives
2 tablespoons extra virgin olive oil
1 tablespoon good-quality wine vinegar

Boil the potatoes whole in salted water until tender—this will take about 20–30 minutes, depending on their size. Keep them whole to keep the centers creamy. Steam the green beans until just cooked.

Finely chop the scallions or shallots and chives and place in a salad bowl. Mix in the olive oil and vinegar.

When the potatoes are cooked, cut in half lengthways, add to the onion mixture, season with salt and pepper and mix well while still hot. Leave the potatoes to infuse in the flavors for 5 minutes, then add the green beans and serve the salad while still warm.

Fiber rating: MEDIUM
Per serving: 3.2g fiber, 146 Calories, 6g fat, 1g saturated fat, 0.5g sodium

Carrot, ginger, and radicchio salad

Serve as part of a selection of salads or with boiled potatoes or warm wholewheat bread for added fiber. There is more fiber if the carrots are unpeeled so I suggest using organic varieties to avoid any chemical sprays on the skin. **Serves 4**

6 medium (11oz.) carrots
7oz. radicchio
⅓ cup pumpkin seeds
Salt and freshly ground black pepper

4 tablespoons sesame oil
1 tablespoon rice vinegar
2 heaping teaspoons finely grated fresh ginger root

Peel and coarsely grate the carrots. Quarter the radicchio, remove the dense white heart and chop finely.

Mix the carrots and radicchio with the pumpkin seeds in a bowl and season with salt and pepper if liked.

Make a dressing with the sesame oil, vinegar, and ginger root. Mix into the salad and serve right away.

Fiber rating: MEDIUM
Per serving: 3.4g fiber, 174 Calories, 14g fat, 2g saturated fat, 0.22g sodium

Broiled peppers with raisins, red onions, and pine nuts

Use red or yellow peppers or a combination of the two in this recipe; green peppers will not work as well. Serve with pita bread or bruschetta (toast rubbed with garlic and extra virgin olive oil) for extra fiber. **Serves 4**

6 large red bell peppers
½ cup pine nuts or slivered almonds
6 tablespoons extra virgin olive oil
1 medium to large red onion, quartered and thinly sliced
1 large garlic clove, crushed
½ cup raisins (or golden raisins)
3 tablespoons sherry vinegar or red wine vinegar
Salt and freshly ground black pepper

Broil the peppers whole until blackened all over, then place in a plastic bag to cool. Remove the skin and cut the peppers into strips, discarding the seeds. Scrape the peppers with a knife if the skins are particularly hard to remove. Do not rinse or you will wash away the flavor. Set aside.

While the peppers are broiling, cook the pine nuts or almonds in 1 tablespoon of the olive oil until light golden brown. Add the onion and garlic and cook slowly until soft. Add the raisins and mix briefly, then add the vinegar. Remove the mixture from the heat, season with salt and pepper, add the remaining oil and leave to soften the raisins for about 5 minutes.

To assemble the salad, place several thin strips of peppers on a plate. Scatter over some of the onion mixture and continue to layer the peppers and onions until all are used up.

Fiber rating: HIGH
Per serving: 5.2g fiber, 370 Calories, 26g fat, 3g saturated fat, 0.51g sodium

Wholewheat pita bread and vegetable salad

Middle Eastern cuisine uses leftover pita bread as the French use dry baguettes: here it soaks up all the lovely juices. Sumac has a sharpness similar to that of lemon zest and is available from Middle Eastern food stores. **Serves 4**

2 wholewheat pita breads
1 large garlic clove, crushed with salt
Juice of 1 large lemon
7 tablespoons extra virgin olive oil
Salt and freshly ground black pepper
1 cup broccoli, cut into florets
1 cup green beans, cut in half
1 medium tomato, cut into large chunks
3 scallions, finely chopped
½ cucumber (9oz.), peeled, halved, and sliced
1 red bell pepper, seeded and sliced
1 small Romaine lettuce, coarsely chopped
4 heaping tablespoons coarsely chopped fresh cilantro
1 tablespoon sumac (optional)

Preheat the oven to 400°F. Heat the pita bread in the oven for about 5–10 minutes, until crisp. Mix the crushed garlic, lemon juice, olive oil, salt and pepper in a large bowl. When the bread is cool enough to handle, break it into small pieces about ¾-inch square and add to the bowl.

Steam or boil the broccoli and green beans until just cooked. Drain well.

Add the tomatoes, scallions, cucumber, red pepper, lettuce, and cilantro to the bread mixture. Add the broccoli and green beans and mix well to coat. Leave to marinate for 10 minutes.

Taste the salad for seasoning and if necessary, add more salt and pepper. Serve as an appetizer, part of a selection of appetizers or as a healthy vegetarian main dish.

Fiber rating: HIGH
Per serving: 6.7g fiber, 466 Calories, 27g fat, 4g saturated fat, 0.6g sodium

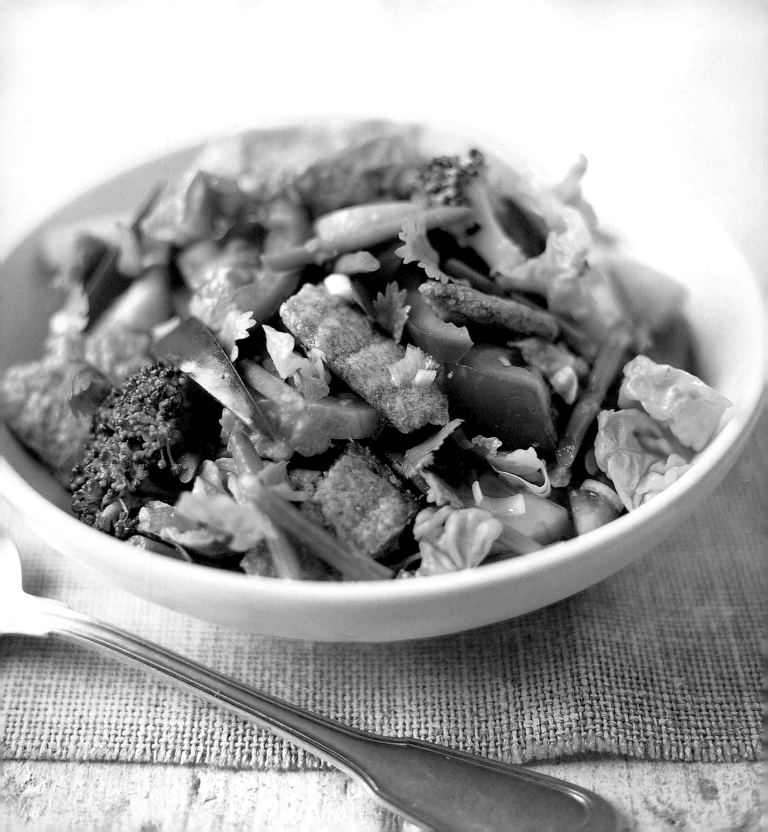

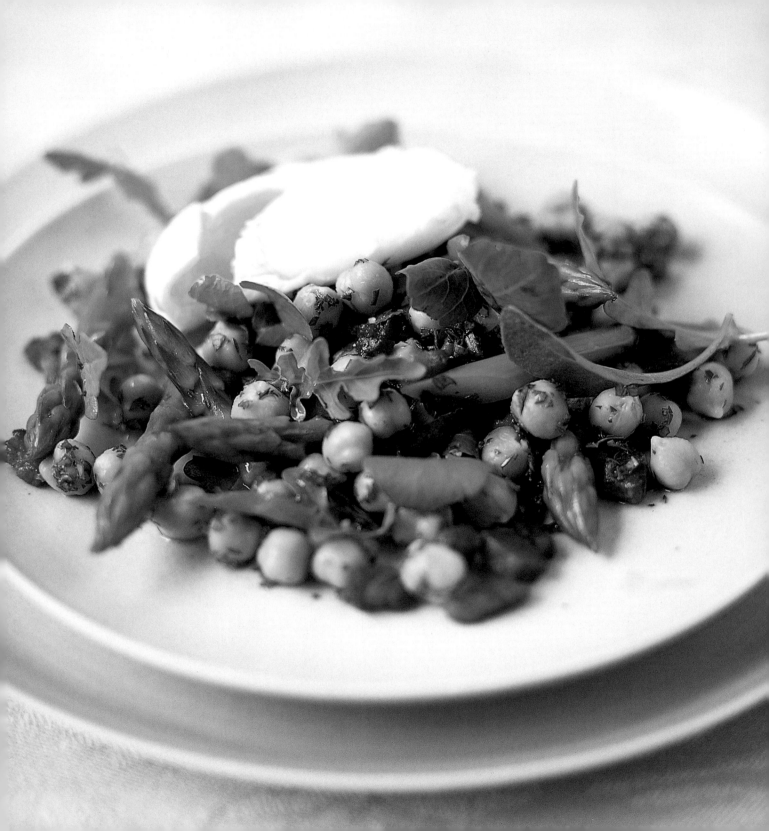

Asparagus, bacon, and chickpea salad

The poached eggs make this salad a meal in itself but can be omitted if you are looking for a lower fat content. Make sure the chickpeas are well rinsed, whether they are cooked from dried or canned, to avoid flatulence. Serves 2

1¼ cups cooked chickpeas	Salt and freshly ground black
2 heaping tablespoons chopped flat-leaf parsley	pepper
	1 bunch asparagus (5 ounces)
1 heaping tablespoon chopped mint	¾ cup smoked bacon lardons or cubes
2 tablespoons lemon juice or sherry vinegar	1 large garlic clove
	2 large handfuls arugula or other salad leaves
3 tablespoons extra virgin olive oil, plus extra for cooking	2 poached eggs (optional)

Rinse the chickpeas well, place in a bowl and add the herbs with 1 tablespoon of the lemon juice or vinegar, 2 tablespoons of the oil, and salt and pepper. Mix well and set aside.

Boil or steam the asparagus for about 3–4 minutes, until just cooked. Drain and set aside.

Fry the bacon over medium-high heat in a dash of olive oil and add the garlic when the bacon is nearly golden and crispy. Set aside.

Place the arugula or other salad leaves in a bowl and add the asparagus and bacon. Pour in the remaining lemon juice or vinegar and the rest of the olive oil. Season with salt and pepper. Divide the salad leaves between two plates and serve with the chickpeas scattered over and a poached egg, if using, on top of each portion.

Fiber rating: HIGH
Per serving, including poached eggs: 5.8g fiber, 401 Calories, 25g fat, 6g saturated fat, 1.68g sodium

Celery root remoulade

This is a French recipe traditionally using mayonnaise, though yogurt is a very good substitute, making it less rich. It is delicious served with smoked duck, chicken breasts or prosciutto ham, and warm crusty bread. Serves 4

1¼ lbs. celery root, peeled and coarsely grated	1½ cups low-fat plain live yogurt
3–4 heaping teaspoons French mustard	Salt and freshly ground black pepper

Place the celery root in a large mixing bowl. Add the mustard and yogurt, season with salt and pepper and mix well to amalgamate. Allow to infuse for at least 15 minutes as this softens the celery root.

Serve as an accompaniment to smoked meats or charcuterie, and warm crusty bread. It tastes even better the next day.

Fiber rating: HIGH
Per serving: 5.6g fiber, 91 Calories, 2g fat, 1g saturated fat, 0.67g sodium

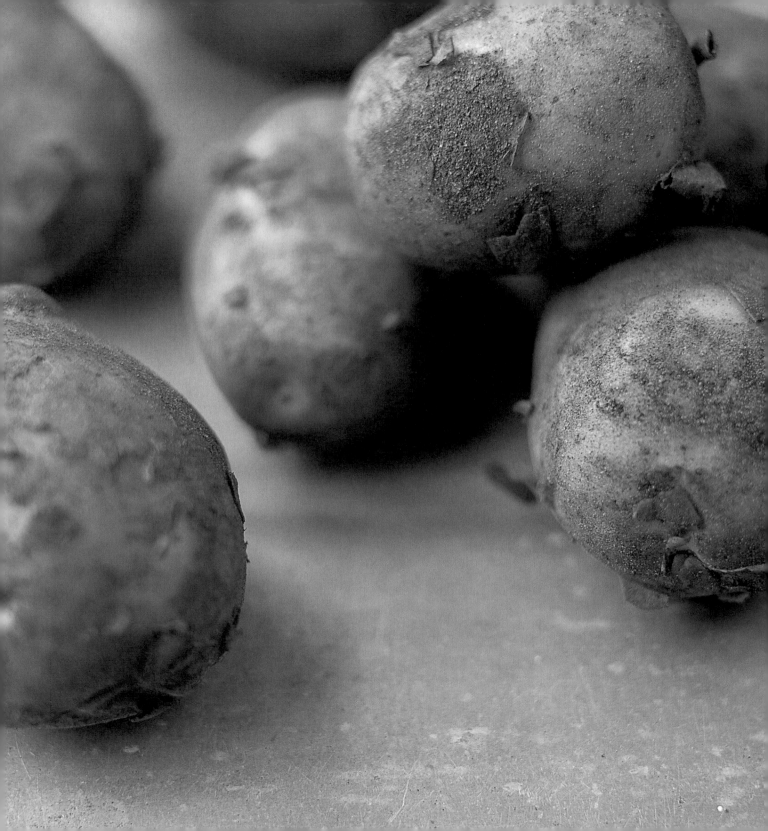

3

Appetizers and Snacks

Asparagus and potato fritatta
As a lunch or snack option this is a yummy alternative to a sandwich. It is also good served with a salad on the side. Other vegetables can be substituted for the asparagus, such as green beans or spinach.

Serves 2 as a main dish or 4 as a light snack

2 medium unpeeled potatoes, cut into 1¼-inch cubes

Salt and freshly ground black pepper

3–4 spears (3oz.) asparagus (trimmed weight)

1 small leek, sliced

2 tablespoons extra virgin olive oil

4 eggs

¼ cup milk

1 tablespoon coarsely chopped basil or parsley

1 tablespoon Parmesan cheese, grated

Salad, to serve (optional)

Boil the potatoes in salted water for about 10 minutes, until just soft. Cut off the tips of the asparagus and slice the stems in half at an angle. Add the asparagus to the potatoes when they are almost cooked and cook for a further 2 minutes. Drain well.

Meanwhile, gently cook the leek in the olive oil in a medium skillet. When it is soft, add the potatoes and asparagus, season with salt and pepper and cook gently for a further 15 minutes, so that the potatoes and asparagus have time to absorb the flavor.

Break the eggs into a bowl and whisk gently with the milk, basil or parsley, salt and pepper.

Preheat the grill to high.

Pour the egg mixture over the vegetables and leave to cook gently for 5 minutes.

Scatter the Parmesan on the top and broil for 1–2 minutes until just set.

Allow to rest for 5 minutes before serving.

Fiber rating: LOW
Per serving (light snack): 1.2g fiber, 199 Calories, 13g fat, 3g saturated fat, 0.42g sodium

Marinated labnah balls
Labnah is a rich, thick yogurt which can be used in a variety of sweet or savory dishes. Here it is rolled into small balls and then marinated in olive oil. Serve with warm wholewheat pita bread and raw vegetables to increase the fiber content. **Makes about 16 balls**

2 cups (18oz.) Greek-style thick live plain yogurt

1 teaspoon salt

2 tablespoons cumin seeds

2 tablespoons paprika

2 tablespoons thyme

1 large red chile, halved or quartered

2 garlic cloves, halved

Sprigs of herbs (e.g., rosemary, thyme, or oregano)

Extra virgin olive oil

Mix the yogurt with the salt, place in a cheesecloth in a strainer over a bowl and leave to drain the whey for about 8 hours or overnight. (If in a hurry, 4 hours is just sufficient.) This thick yogurt cheese is then ready to be used in cooking savory and sweet dishes.

To make the labnah balls, ensure the yogurt is properly drained and of a dense texture for best results. Roll the yogurt into 1¼-inch balls, then roll in the cumin seeds, paprika, and thyme. Place in a bowl or sterilized jelly jar, and add the red chile, garlic, and sprigs of herbs, and cover with olive oil to marinate.

They keep for a couple of weeks in the fridge and are perfect to eat when your cupboard looks bare: serve them on toast, smeared on broiled meats, or in sandwiches as a healthy alternative to mayonnaise or cream cheese.

Fiber rating: LOW
Per serving (2 labnah balls): 0g fiber, 86 Calories, 8g fat, 3g saturated fat, 0.29g sodium

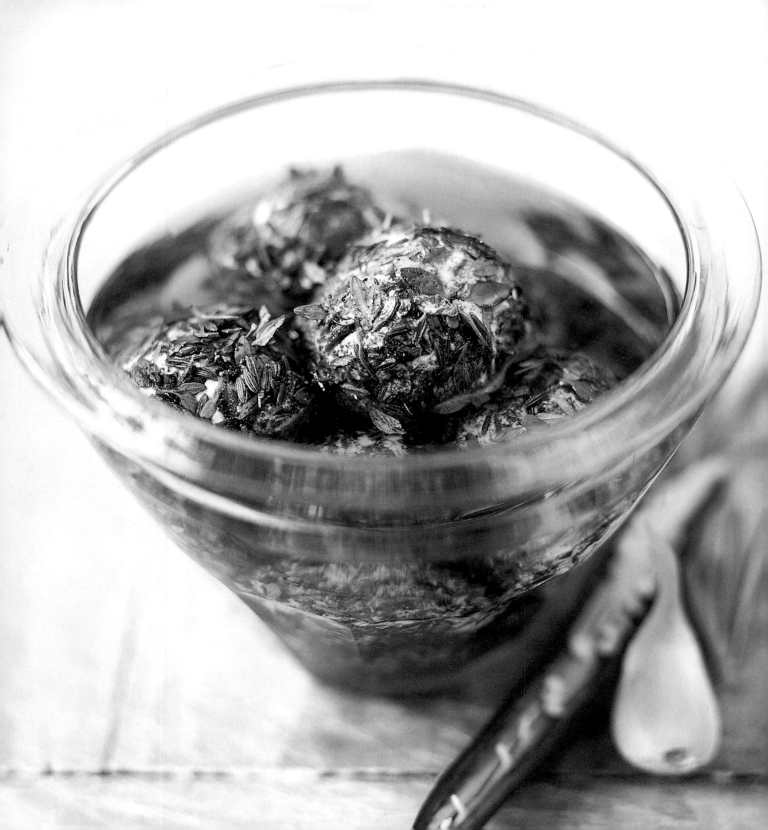

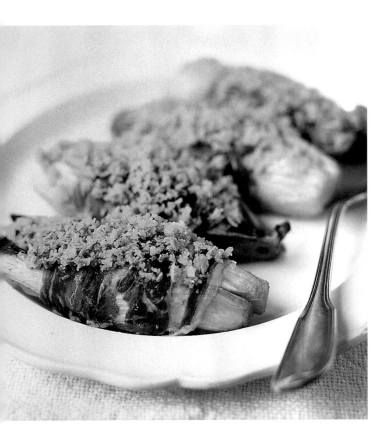

Baked endive wrapped in prosciutto

Endive is sometimes known as chicory. This is a simple dish to serve on its own with some bread to mop up the juices. It's also good with baked white fish or a broiled lamb or pork chop.

Serves 4

4 large heads endive bulbs

8 large basil leaves

3½ oz. prosciutto or speck, thinly sliced

1 large garlic clove, finely chopped

½ cup wholewheat or white breadcrumbs

5 tablespoons Parmesan cheese, grated

1 tablespoon extra virgin olive oil

Freshly ground black pepper

1 cup chicken stock

Preheat the oven to 375°F.

Cut the endive in half lengthwise. Place a basil leaf on each half and wrap a slice of prociutto around the endive. Place in a gratin dish about 8 x 10 inches so that they fit snugly in one layer.

Mix the garlic with the breadcrumbs, Parmesan, olive oil, and pepper. (The oil helps to crisp the breadcrumbs, making a crunchy topping). Scatter over the endive.

Pour the stock carefully into the dish down one side—avoid soaking the breadcrumbs. It should come about halfway up the endive. Cover with aluminum foil and bake for 45 minutes. Remove the foil and cook a further 30 minutes, until the endive is soft at the thickest end.

Take the dish out of the oven and allow to rest for at least 15 minutes before serving.

Fiber rating: LOW

Per serving, with wholewheat breadcrumbs: 2.8g fiber, 141 Calories, 8g fat, 3g saturated fat, 0.87g sodium

Stuffed vine leaves

A combination of red rice and barley is used to increase the fiber content of this dish. Vine leaves are often used in Mediterranean countries, where they grow in abundance. If using fresh vine leaves, blanch in salted water for 2 minutes and drain before stuffing. **Serves 6**

½ cup pine nuts

3 tablespoons extra virgin olive oil

1 large onion, finely chopped

2 garlic cloves, finely chopped

¾ cup mixture of red rice and barley

⅓ cup raisins

1 teaspoon ground allspice

Salt and freshly ground black pepper

4 tablespoons chopped mint

9-oz. packet vine leaves in salt water

9oz. fennel bulb, cut into thin wedges or slices

Low-fat plain live yogurt, to serve (optional)

Gently cook the pine nuts in 2 tablespoons of the oil, then add the onion and garlic and cook for about 10 minutes until the onion is soft and the pine nuts golden. Add the rice and barley, raisins, and allspice, season with salt and pepper and mix briefly.

Pour over 2½ cups hot water, cover with a lid and cook for 40 minutes. Remove the lid and, if there is still some water left, reduce until the mixture is dry. Spoon into a bowl and add the chopped mint.

Remove the vine leaves from the packet, cover with boiling water and leave to soak for 5 minutes. Drain well.

Pour the remaining oil into an ovenproof dish or heavy saucepan, about 9 inches wide. Scatter over the fennel pieces so that they cover the base.

Preheat the oven, if using, to 350°F.

Place a vine leaf on a work surface, with the rough side facing up. Place 1 level tablespoon of the rice filling in the middle of the leaf (depending on the size), fold over from the bottom, folding the sides into the middle as you go, and roll up tightly to keep it sealed. Place on top of the fennel, folded side down. Repeat until all the filling is used and fit the stuffed leaves snugly into the dish or pan in one layer so that they don't open up when cooking. If your dish or pan is not wide enough for one layer, arrange another layer on top, drizzling a little olive oil between the layers.

Pour in enough water to come three-quarters of the way up the vine leaves. Cover with a lid or aluminum foil and place in the oven for 1 hour, or simmer very gently on the stove for 45 minutes. When cooking on the stove the water might evaporate, but that is ok—just add a dash more if not cooked through.

Remove from the heat and leave uncovered to cool. Serve warm or at room temperature with a dollop of yogurt.

Fiber rating: MEDIUM

Per serving not including yogurt: 3.8g fiber, 200 Calories, 12g fat, 1g saturated fat, 1.13g sodium

Dukkah (Egyptian nut dip) *Eat with high-fiber flatbread if you want to make this into a high-fiber recipe; dunking it in extra virgin olive oil will make the dukkah stick to it. Delicious with thick-set yogurt or labnah and raw vegetables such as radishes, scallions, and tomatoes.* **Serves 6**

8½ oz. cooked chickpeas, rinsed and drained
1 cup blanched hazelnuts
1¼ cups sesame seeds
2 heaping tablespoons coriander seeds
1 tablespoon cumin seeds
1 heaping teaspoon sea salt
1 heaping teaspoon freshly ground black pepper

Preheat the oven to 350°F. Place the chickpeas on a roasting sheet in the oven and cook for about 45 minutes until dry and slightly crunchy. Meanwhile, cook the hazelnuts and sesame seeds on separate baking sheets in the oven for about 15 minutes, until both are golden brown. Set aside and leave to cool.

Dry-roast the coriander and then the cumin seeds in a skillet on a medium heat for a few minutes until they start to color very slightly and give off a mild aroma. Watch them carefully as they can burn very easily.

Grind the spices first, using a mortar and pestle for best results. (A solid bowl and the end of a rolling pin make a good substitute.) Place the spices in a bowl. It might be easier to grind in batches. Then grind half the sesame seeds and add the rest whole to the spices. Coarsely grind the hazelnuts and finally the chickpeas, so they keep some texture.

Mix the ground ingredients together and add the salt and pepper. Taste to check for correct seasoning and adjust as necessary.

Serve the dukkah as suggested above. It will keep for several weeks in an airtight container.

Fiber rating: MEDIUM
Per serving: 4g fiber, 254 Calories, 22g fat, 2g saturated fat, 0.61g sodium

Bruschetta with chard, borlotti beans, and anchovy sauce *A great Italian recipe, ideal for non-meat eaters. Some chard has large white stalks, but these can be used as well in the recipe: boil for longer and cut into small pieces.* **Serves 4**

14oz. chard leaves
14-oz. can borlotti or cannellini beans, drained and rinsed
4 large slices sourdough bread
Salt and freshly ground black pepper
1 garlic clove

For the anchovy sauce
2-oz. can anchovies in oil, drained, or jar of salted anchovies, rinsed and drained
1 tablespoon chopped rosemary
2 tablespoons lemon juice
3½ tablespoons extra virgin olive oil
Freshly ground black pepper

To make the anchovy sauce, put the anchovies and rosemary in a food processor with the lemon juice. Mix together and slowly add the olive oil. (You can also make the sauce by hand using a mortar and pestle.) Taste to see if you need to add more oil or lemon juice, if you prefer a milder anchovy flavor. Season with pepper and set aside. If the sauce separates, just give it a good stir before serving—it is not meant to be a mayonnaise.

Cook the chard in boiling water until tender. Drain and set aside. Place the chard and beans in separate bowls and add ½ tablespoon of the anchovy sauce to each. Mix and season with salt and pepper.

Toast the bread and, while it is still hot, rub on both sides with the cut side of the garlic. Place the bruschetta on plates, place the chard on top, scatter over the beans and finally drizzle over the remaining anchovy sauce. Serve right away.

Fiber rating: MEDIUM
Per serving: 4.3g fiber, 331 Calories, 15g fat, 2g saturated fat, 1.15g sodium

Shrimp on toast

For best results try to find the tiny shrimps which the French call "grey shrimp" or which the English use in potted shrimp recipes. You could serve these as nibbles at a party using bite-sized pieces of toast. **Serves 2 as an appetizer or light snack**

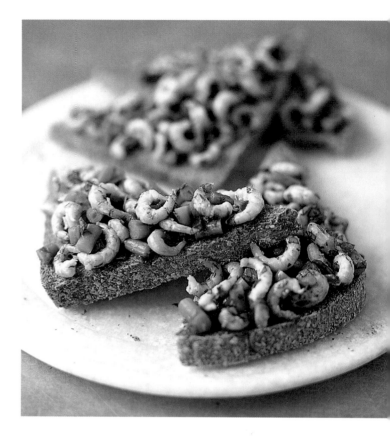

1 cup cooked shrimp

1 cup cooked green beans, diced

2 tablespoons coarsely chopped flat-leaf parsley

½ broiled or raw red pepper or ½ large mild red chile, seeded and diced

Juice of ½ lemon

3 tablespoons extra virgin olive oil

Freshly ground black pepper

2 slices wholewheat bread

1 garlic clove

Salad leaves, such as arugula (optional)

Rinse the shrimp and dry well on kitchen paper towels. Mix the shrimp with the diced beans, chopped parsley, diced chile or pepper, lemon juice, 1 tablespoon of the extra virgin olive oil, and pepper. Leave to marinate for a few minutes.

Toast the bread and, while it is still warm, rub with the cut side of the garlic. Place the toasts on plates on top of some salad leaves, if using, and spoon over the shrimp mixture. **Finally** drizzle over the remaining oil and serve right away.

Fiber rating: MEDIUM
Per serving: 3.8g fiber, 300 Calories, 18g fat, 3g saturated fat, 0.7g sodium

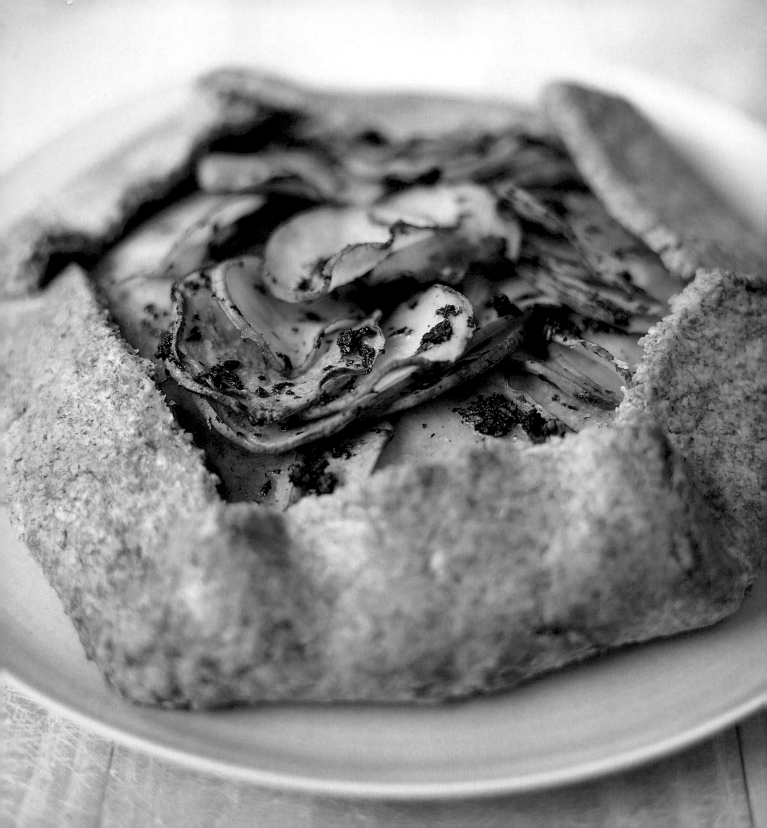

Potato galette with wholewheat pastry

A galette is an open pastry tart. This simple yet sophisticated dish needs just a green salad to accompany it. As with all pastry dishes, this is a relatively high-fat recipe, so is best avoided if you are on a low-fat diet. **Serves 4 as main, 6 as appetizer**

14oz. ready-made wholewheat pastry

2 medium baking potatoes, unpeeled

2 medium sweet potatoes, unpeeled

Salt and freshly ground black pepper

2 tablespoons chopped sage

4 tablespoons extra virgin olive oil

1 garlic clove, smashed with salt into a pulp

3 heaping teaspoons mushroom and truffle paste

1 egg yolk, mixed with 1 tablespoon milk for the egg wash

On a floured work surface, roll out the pastry into a rough square about 14 inches across and ⅛-inch thick. Move the pastry round by a quarter turn with each roll to prevent it from sticking to the work surface and to create a uniform shape. Place a sheet of aluminum foil on a board or large plate, place the pastry on it and chill for 15 minutes.

Place a baking sheet in the oven and preheat to 400°F. Thinly slice the potatoes and sweet potatoes. Place the slices in a bowl and season with salt and pepper. Mix in the sage, oil, crushed garlic, and truffle paste.

Remove the pastry from the fridge and trim into a 13-inch circle. Arrange the potato mixture in the middle, leaving a 2-inch border around the edges. Fold up the sides of the pastry in about five turns, encasing the potatoes but leaving the center showing.

Glaze the pastry edges with egg wash and lift the pastry, still on the foil, onto the warmed baking sheet. Bake for 30 minutes until the pastry is light golden brown. Turn the heat down to 350°F and cover the potato center with a little sheet of aluminum foil. Cook for a further 30 minutes, then remove from the oven, leave to rest for at least 15 minutes, and serve.

Fiber rating: HIGH
Per serving (appetizer): 6.7g fiber, 517 Calories, 31g fat, 8g saturated fat, 0.61g sodium

Avocado, fennel, and cucumber relish with flatbread

This relish works well served with a selection of other salads. The high fiber content of this recipe comes from the wholewheat pita bread, so use white pita bread if you need to decrease the fiber. **Serves 4**

½ large cucumber

1 teaspoon sea salt

1 teaspoon fennel seeds, ground or 7-oz. bulb fennel

1 ripe avocado

1 tablespoon tahini or toasted sesame seeds

1 garlic clove, crushed with salt

2 tablespoons coarsely chopped tarragon

3 heaping tablespoons low-fat plain live yogurt

Freshly ground black pepper

1 tablespoon lemon juice (optional)

4 large wholewheat pita or flatbread, to serve

Peel the cucumber and slice in half lengthwise. Remove the seeds with a teaspoon, slice into thin strips and chop finely. Place the cucumber pieces in a colander and mix with the salt. Leave to drain for 15 minutes. This releases some of the liquid from the cucumber, making the relish less watery. Squeeze the cucumber between your hands to release the remaining juices and place in a bowl.

Add the ground fennel to the cucumber. If using fresh fennel, trim any green fronds and chop them finely. Cut out and discard the tough heart and chop the rest into small pieces. Add to the cucumber along with the chopped fronds. Peel, pit and coarsely chop the avocado and add to the bowl. You could use a food processor to do the chopping if preferred.

Stir the tahini paste well, as it tends to separate if left to stand, then add it or the sesame seeds to the bowl. Add the crushed garlic, tarragon, and yogurt, season with pepper and mix well.

Taste and add more salt if needed—though enough may have already been added with the garlic and cucumber. Add the lemon juice if the yogurt used is not very tart.

Fiber rating: HIGH
Per serving including bread: 7.3g fiber, 403 Calories, 14g fat, 2g saturated fat, 0.95g sodium

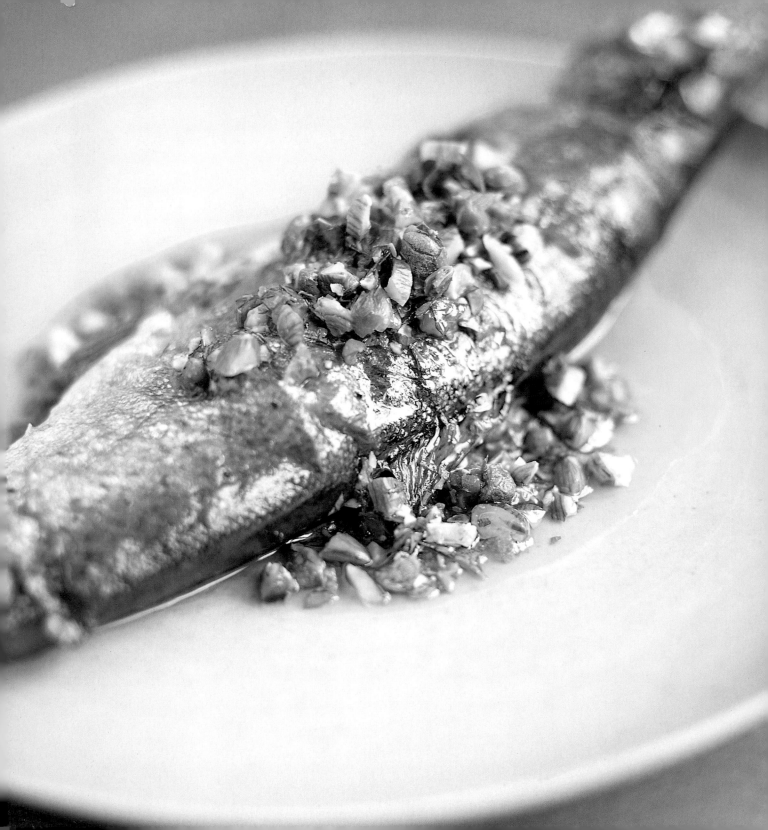

4

Fish

Sardine kofta with tomatoes and spices
This is a dish from Morocco where really fresh sardines are plentiful. You could try substituting any oily fish such as mackerel or grey mullet; the freshness of the fish is more important than the type. Serve with warm pita bread and salad. **Serves 4**

1lb. fresh sardine fillets	2 heaping tablespoons
1 heaping teaspoon cumin seeds	coarsely chopped fresh
1 heaping teaspoon cilantro	cilantro
seeds	Salt and freshly ground black
½ large chile, chopped	pepper
(optional)	2 tablespoons extra virgin
2 garlic cloves, chopped	olive oil
2 tablespoons fresh	14-oz. can chopped tomatoes
breadcrumbs, wholewheat	1 small lemon, cut into thin
or plain	slices

Remove any large bones remaining in the sardine fillets and rinse to clean away any scales or blood. Don't worry about small bones down the middle of the fish. Drain on paper towels.
Grind the cumin and cilantro seeds in a spice grinder or mortar and pestle.
Place the fish in a food processor with the ground cumin and coriander, the chile, if using, garlic, breadcrumbs, and half the cilantro. Season well with salt and pepper and mix thoroughly.
Preheat the oven to 300°F. Roll the sardine mixture into about 20 x 1-oz. balls. Set aside.
Heat the olive oil in a large ovenproof sauté pan (or tagine), add the tomatoes, and cook until reduced, stirring periodically to prevent them burning on the base of the pan. Add the sardine balls and cook on a medium-high heat for 1 minute. Turn the balls over; add 2 tablespoons water so that the tomatoes are not too dry. Lay the lemon slices on top of the balls; cover the pan with a lid and place in the oven for 10 minutes.
Remove the sardine kofta from the oven and scatter with the remaining fresh cilantro. Serve hot or at room temperature.

Fiber rating: LOW
Per serving: 1g fiber, 276 Calories, 16g fat, 4g saturated fat, 0.72g sodium

Broiled trout with almonds
It is always good to revisit old classics and make them healthy. Serve with a watercress and green bean salad and boiled new potatoes for added fiber. The fish can also be griddled or baked (see picture on page 82). **Serves 2**

Drizzle of olive oil, for greasing	¼ cup almonds, roasted in a
4 tablespoons extra virgin	medium oven for about
olive oil	10 minutes, then finely
2 tablespoons lemon juice or	chopped
white wine vinegar	Salt and freshly ground black
2 heaping tablespoons coarsely	pepper
chopped flat-leaf parsley	2 x 7-oz. whole trout, cleaned
1 heaping tablespoon capers,	and gutted
rinsed and finely chopped	

Preheat the grill to high. Cover the grill sheet with aluminum foil and drizzle over a little oil so the fish doesn't stick when cooking. Mix the olive oil with the lemon juice or vinegar, parsley, capers, and almonds. Season with salt and pepper, and set aside. This can be prepared in advance.
Cook the fish for about 4 minutes on each side. Reduce the heat or lower the shelf if the skin is starting to burn before the fish is cooked. Check that it is ready by lifting a little of the flesh by the middle fin. If the flesh is just cooked through to the bone, turn the trout over to hide the incision and serve right away with the almond salsa.
If baking the fish, preheat the oven to 400°F, and cook for about 10–15 minutes until the eye is opaque and the flesh just firm.

Fiber rating: LOW
Per serving: 1.4g fiber, 503 Calories, 37g fat, 4g saturated fat, 0.21g sodium

Mussel, saffron, and yogurt stew

*I wanted to include a shellfish recipe and this is an interesting way
to cook mussels. The recipe is low in fiber but if you served some
lentils or a chickpea salad with it the fiber would be increased.*

Serves 6

4½ lbs. mussels

½ cup brown or white rice

2 large pinches of saffron
strands

3½ tablespoons dry white
vermouth or sherry

⅓ cup white wine

1 large red onion, finely
chopped

1 large carrot, finely chopped

2 large garlic cloves

3 tablespoons extra virgin
olive oil

¾ cup Greek-style yogurt, or
low-fat plain yogurt mixed
with 1 heaping teaspoon
cornstarch

1 small bunch cilantro or dill,
coarsely chopped

Make sure the mussels are debearded and properly cleaned.
Wash them in several changes of water and drain.

Cook the rice in boiling water to cover with a pinch of
saffron for about 10 minutes, or longer for brown rice, until
the water has evaporated and the rice is just tender. Set aside
to steam, covered with a lid. Soak the remaining saffron in the
vermouth or sherry.

Heat a large saucepan with a tight-fitting lid. Unless you have
a very big pan, cook the mussels in batches, making sure they
cover the base of the pan—don't put in too many at once or
they won't cook evenly. Throw the mussels in with some of
the wine, cover and cook for about 2 minutes. Lift the lid after
1 minute and check that the mussels are cooking quickly and
starting to open. Stir well, cover again and cook for another
1–2 minutes, depending on their size. Cook just until the
shells open – discard any that fail to open. Pour into a colander
that is resting inside a bowl to collect the juices. Rinse the pan
briefly and repeat until all mussels are cooked. Remove the
shells once cool, discarding the shells. Pour the cooking juices
into a container, discarding the sediment, and set aside.

Rinse the pan again before cooking the base of the stew.
Gently cook the onion, carrot, and garlic in the olive oil for
10 minutes until they are soft and the onion is transparent.
Add the saffron and vermouth and bring to a boil. Reduce for
a minute or two. Add the reserved cooking liquid and the
yogurt mixed with cornstarch (the latter prevents it
separating). Bring to a simmer, then add the mussels and half
the chopped herb. Remove from the heat.

Divide the rice between six warmed bowls and pour the stew
on top. Sprinkle with the remaining herb and serve right away.

Fiber rating: LOW
Per serving with brown rice: 1.3g fiber, 251 Calories, 12g fat,
3g saturated fat, 0.37g sodium

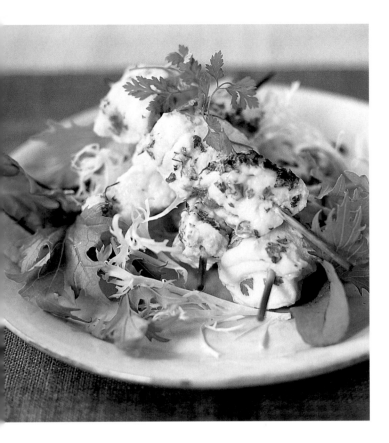

Monkfish kebabs marinated with herbs and yogurt

The yogurt helps to tenderize the fish. Salmon can be used instead of monkfish if you like. Serve with brown rice, or lentils and braised spinach, to increase the fiber content. **Serves 4**

1¼ lbs. monkfish fillet, cut into 1-inch cubes

¾ cup set low-fat plain yogurt

2 tablespoons chervil or dill, coarsely chopped

Salt and freshly ground black pepper

Skewers

Mix the fish cubes in a bowl with the yogurt and half the chervil. Season with salt and pepper and leave to marinate. Preheat the grill to high.

Place the fish pieces on skewers or line them in rows on a baking sheet, smearing over any excess yogurt from the bowl.

Cook for about 5–10 minutes, depending on the size of the cubes of fish and the heat of the grill. They should be just firm to the touch.

Serve the kebabs on a bed of rice or salad if you like, pour over the cooking juices and scatter over the remaining chervil or dill for a fresh taste.

Fiber rating: LOW

Per serving: 0g fiber, 157 Calories, 6g fat, 3g saturated fat, 0.35g sodium

Syrian stuffed fish with rice and tamarind

Any round fish that is fresh will work in this recipe. The tartness of tamarind combines well with the sweetness of the figs. Serve with spinach or green beans for added fiber.

Serves 6

3lbs. 5oz. sea bass, bream or other round fish large enough to stuff

2 tablespoons extra virgin olive oil, plus extra for greasing

½ cup pine nuts

½ cup almonds, coarsely chopped

1 medium red onion, finely chopped

2 garlic cloves, chopped

⅔ cup dried figs, chopped

¾ cup brown or white basmati rice

Salt and freshly ground black pepper

Small pinch of saffron, soaked in 1 tablespoon water

Grated zest and juice of large lime

2 heaping teaspoons grated fresh ginger root

2 tablespoons tamarind paste

2 tablespoons brown sugar

Chopped cilantro, to serve

Ask the fish merchant to scale, gut, and clean the fish. Rinse the fish just before cooking to remove any remaining blood. Set aside on kitchen paper towels to drain.

Pour the olive oil into a large saucepan, add the pine nuts and almonds and cook briefly until they turn a light golden brown. Add the onion and garlic, turn the heat down to low and continue cooking for a further 10 minutes until the onion is soft. Add the figs, rice, and some salt, stir briefly, then add the saffron and enough water just to cover the rice if using white rice, a little more if using brown. Bring to a boil and simmer for about 10 minutes for white rice and 30 minutes for brown. Leave covered for 10 minutes off the heat. The rice should be just cooked. Remove the lid and, if there is any water left, evaporate until dry. Stir in the lime zest. Leave to cool completely unless cooking the fish immediately.

Preheat the oven with a baking sheet to 400°F.

In a small saucepan, heat the lime juice, ginger root, tamarind, sugar and about 2 tablespoons water. Stir and simmer briefly until the sugar has dissolved. Set aside.

Prepare a piece of aluminum foil big enough to seal the fish in and drizzle a little olive oil in the middle so the fish doesn't stick. Place the fish on the foil and place half the tamarind sauce in the belly. Stuff as much of the rice as possible into the fish, placing the rest next to it as it will be all sealed in the foil. Pour the remaining tamarind sauce on top of the fish. Season with salt and pepper. Fold up the sides of the foil, sealing all the edges well. Remove the heated baking sheet from the oven and carefully place the fish on it. Cook the fish in the oven for about 20 minutes. If you have prepared the rice in advance and it is cold, allow a further 10 minutes. The fish is cooked when the eye looks opaque or the color of poached eggs.

To serve, place the fish on an oval plate—it should slide easily off the aluminum foil if well greased. Sprinkle over some cilantro for color.

Fiber rating: LOW

Per serving with brown rice: 2.8g fiber, 591 Calories, 25g fat, 5g saturated fat, 0.51g sodium

Mackerel simmered in miso soup

This Japanese dish uses miso to give a delicious nutty, salty flavor. Dashi is a fish stock made with bonito (dried tuna) flakes. Try using other oily fish if good fresh mackerel are not available. Serve with steamed snow peas and brown and white rice. **Serves 4**

4 mackerel fillets, about 14oz. total weight
⅛-oz. packet bonito flakes (packet miso soup or fish stock can be substituted)
2 tablespoons sake
2 tablespoons mirin or dry white vermouth
1 teaspoon sugar
1 small piece fresh ginger root, peeled and cut into 16 very thin slivers
1 heaping tablespoon miso paste
2 thin scallions, thinly sliced

Wash and clean the mackerel fillets and dry on paper towels.
Make the dashi (fish stock) by placing the bonito flakes in a measuring cup and pouring ¾ cup boiling water over them. Leave for 5 minutes and drain, discarding the bonito flakes. (A thrifty Japanese would reuse the bonito flakes, mixing them with white rice and sesame seeds or with wilted spinach). Mix in the sake, mirin or vermouth, and sugar.
Warm a serving dish. Place 4 thin slivers of ginger root on top of each mackerel fillet. Pour the dashi into a large sauté pan or skillet and add the mackerel fillets. Bring the liquid just to a boil, cover with a lid and cook the fish for 3–4 minutes, depending on size, until it is just firm and cooked.
Remove the mackerel fillets from the pan, place on the warmed serving dish and keep warm. Add the miso to the cooking liquid and bring to a boil. Simmer for a couple of minutes to reduce a little. Add the sliced scallions and pour the sauce over the mackerel. Serve right away with rice and snow peas.

Fiber rating: LOW
Per serving: 0.1g fiber, 251 Calories, 16g fat, 3g saturated fat, 0.17g sodium

Baked fish parcels with julienne of vegetables
An attractive dinner party recipe. I suggest you use thin pieces of fish rather than thick as the bright color of the vegetables will diminish if cooked for too long. Serve with lentils, potatoes with skins, or borlotti beans to increase the fiber. **Serves 4**

2 medium leeks, thinly sliced
3 tablespoons sunflower oil
1 large garlic clove, grated
1 heaping teaspoon grated fresh ginger
2 medium carrots, coarsely grated
2 cups (5oz.) snow peas, thinly sliced
2 tablespoons chopped tarragon
4 x 3½-oz. fillets white fish, e.g., cod, bream, monkfish
4 tablespoons dry white vermouth or white wine

Place a large baking sheet in the oven and preheat to 400°F.
Cook the leeks in 1 tablespoon of the sunflower oil on medium-high heat for 2 minutes. Stir frequently to prevent browning. Once softened, add the ginger root and garlic and cook for a further minute. Remove from the heat and stir in the carrots, snow peas, and tarragon. Season if liked and set aside.
Cut 4 large sheets of aluminum foil about 15½ inches square. Drizzle ½ tablespoon of oil three-quarters of the way up each piece of foil (so that when folded, this becomes the middle of the parcel). Divide the vegetables evenly between the foil squares, placing them on the oil. Top with a fillet of fish and season with salt and pepper. Pour 1 tablespoon vermouth over each fillet and fold up the foil. Seal by carefully folding over both sides several times and pressing down well. Finally fold over the top several times so that the fish is completely sealed.
Place the fish parcels on the preheated baking sheet, overlapping the ends of the parcels if necessary. Cook in the oven for 10–15 minutes, depending on the thickness of the fish. To check that the fish is cooked, carefully unfold one, taking care not to let the steam burn you.
Transfer the fish parcels to serving plates and let your guests open them up themselves. Bear in mind that they will carry on cooking if not opened immediately.

Fiber rating: LOW
Per serving: 2.6g fiber, 200 Calories, 9g fat, 1g saturated fat, 0.07g sodium

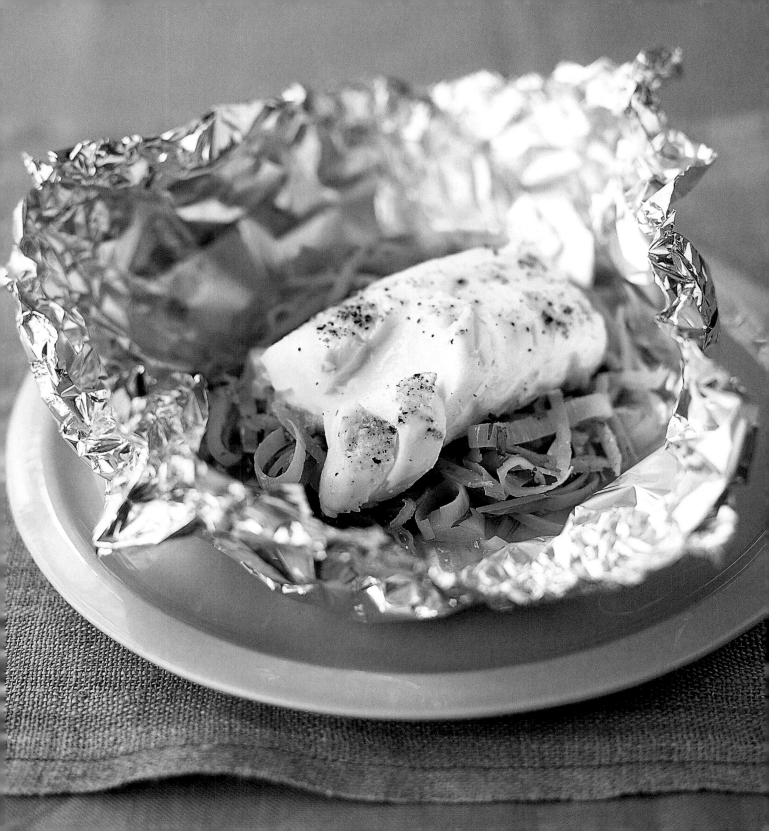

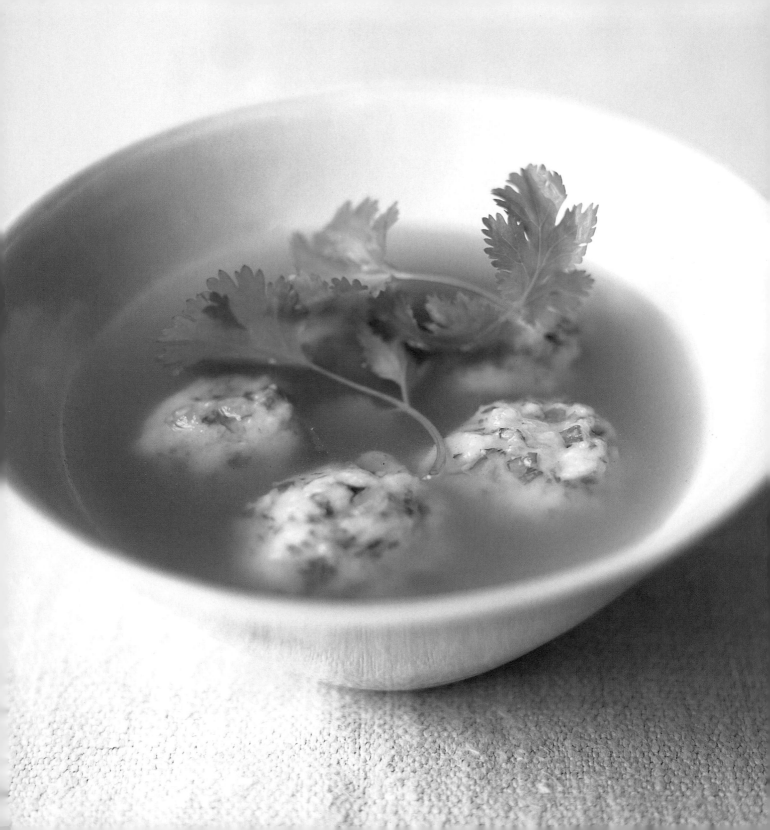

Thai shrimp balls in lemon grass fish broth

Any firm white fish can be substituted for shrimp if you prefer. Choose noodles and vegetables with appropriate fiber levels to serve with. Snow peas work particularly well with this dish. **Serves 4**

12oz. unpeeled raw shrimp (10oz. peeled weight)

14 lime leaves

2 lemon grass sticks, cut into chunks

2 heaping tablespoons coarsely chopped Thai basil or cilantro

2 tablespoons Thai fish sauce

2 teaspoons cornstarch

2 egg whites

½ cup green beans, finely chopped into discs

1 tablespoon coarsely chopped galangal (optional)

Few cilantro sprigs, for garnishing

Peel the shrimp, placing the shrimp shells in a saucepan. Cover with 4 cups water, 4 of the lime leaves and 1 of the lemon grass sticks. Bring to a boil and simmer for 30 minutes. Drain into a measuring cup to make sure you have about 2 cups tasty shrimp broth. Rinse the pan and place the shrimp stock back in the pan, discarding any sediment at the bottom. Set aside.

Devein the shrimp, removing the thin black food sac down the middle, rinse and drain well on kitchen paper towels. Remove the central vein from 6 of the lime leaves and discard; chop the leaves. Place the shrimp and lime leaves in a food processor and add the basil or cilantro, fish sauce, cornstarch and egg whites. Blend well, stir in the green beans and set aside to rest. Test whether the mixture has enough seasoning by cooking a little ball of it in some of the stock. Then, using your hands, form the mixture into 20 balls.

Bring the shrimp stock back to a boil, add the remaining lime leaves, the remaining lemon grass, and the galangal, if using. Bring to a boil again and simmer for a few minutes. Remove the lemon grass and lime leaves with a slotted spoon. Add the shrimp balls to the stock, cooking as many as you can at one time. Cook for 4 minutes, turning over halfway through.

Warm four bowls and divide the fish balls between them. Pour the broth over and scatter a few sprigs of cilantro on top. Serve right away.

Fiber rating: LOW

Per serving: 0g fiber, 81 Calories, 1g fat, 0g saturated fat, 0.76g sodium

Broiled swordfish with cannellini bean salad

Any fish can be used in this recipe, just as long as it is fresh. Other beans can be used in the salad if necessary. Basil mayonnaise is a delicious accompaniment if you don't mind the fat content. **Serves 4**

4 x 3½oz. swordfish steaks
2 heaping tablespoons finely chopped basil
2 tablespoons extra virgin olive oil, plus extra for the fish
Salt and freshly ground black pepper
4 lemon wedges

For the bean salad
2 tablespoons extra virgin olive oil
6-oz. bulb fennel, thinly sliced
2 red bell peppers, seeded and thinly sliced
1 large garlic clove, chopped
Salt and freshly ground black pepper
14-oz. can cannellini beans, drained and rinsed
2 large handfuls baby spinach, washed

To make the salad, heat the oil in a saucepan and add the fennel, red peppers, garlic, and salt and pepper. Cook over a medium heat, covered with a lid, for about 20 minutes, stirring periodically until the vegetables are soft.

Add the beans and cook for a further minute. Add the spinach, stirring until it just wilts. This can be served hot or cold.

To cook the fish, heat a griddle until hot. Finely chop the basil, mix with the oil and season with salt and pepper. Set aside. Lightly oil the fish and cook for about 2–3 minutes, depending on its thickness. Season with salt and pepper.

Serve the bean salad with the fish on top. Drizzle over the basil and serve with a wedge of lemon to squeeze over the fish.

Fiber rating: MEDIUM
Per serving: 3.1g fiber, 249 Calories, 16g fat, 3g saturated fat, 0.39g sodium

Baked salmon with lentils and spinach

If you haven't tried lentils with salmon before, you may be surprised at how well they complement one another. Lentils are a good source of fiber and can be easily prepared in advance. **Serves 4**

¾ cup green or Puy lentils
1 large garlic clove, quartered
2 tablespoons extra virgin olive oil, plus extra for the fish
3½ oz. spinach, coarsely chopped
4 x 5oz. salmon fillets
Salt and freshly ground black pepper

⅔ cup low-fat Greek style yogurt
To serve
4 medium tomatoes, halved and roasted, or 2 large broiled and skinned red bell peppers, cut into strips

Place the lentils in a saucepan and cover generously with water. Add the garlic and 1 tablespoon of the oil and bring to a boil. Reduce the heat and simmer for 30 minutes, until the lentils are just soft. Drain well, remove the skin from the garlic and set aside.

Rinse the saucepan to remove any lentil sediment on the sides. Add the remaining oil to the pan along with the spinach leaves. Cook the spinach gently for a few minutes until it just wilts. Add the drained cooked lentils and garlic and season with salt and pepper, mixing well. Set aside.

Heat a griddle or grill and very lightly smear the fish with a little oil. Season with salt and pepper and cook for about 5–7 minutes on each side, depending on the thickness, until just cooked. Salmon is one fish that can be served slightly rare.

Rewarm the lentils and stir in the yogurt. Remove immediately from the heat and serve right away. The yogurt will separate if overheated.

Place the lentils on warmed plates and serve the salmon on top with roasted tomatoes or broiled peppers to add extra sweetness.

Fiber rating: MEDIUM
Per serving: 4.3g fiber, 487 Calories, 25g fat, 4g saturated fat, 0.63g sodium

Salmon wrapped in vine leaves
with couscous

If only little cans of very fiery harissa are available, mix with 1 large grilled red pepper, finely chopped, and ½ teaspoon each ground cumin and coriander seeds. Increase the fiber content if needed with some high-fiber vegetables. **Serves 4**

16 vine leaves (3½oz.) in salted water (can be omitted if unavailable)

4 x 5-oz. salmon fillets (cod can be substituted)

Salt and freshly ground black pepper

1 small bunch thyme

Drizzle of olive oil

For the couscous

5-oz. bulb fennel, finely chopped and fronds (if any) reserved

1 cup green beans, finely chopped

2 garlic cloves, chopped

2 tablespoons extra virgin olive oil

Salt and freshly ground black pepper

¼ cup raisins

1 teaspoon fennel seeds, ground

½ teaspoon ground cinnamon

¾ cup couscous

2 tablespoons coarsely chopped flat-leaf parsley

1 tablespoon coarsely chopped mint

2 heaping tablespoons good-quality harissa (chile) sauce

1 lemon, cut into wedges

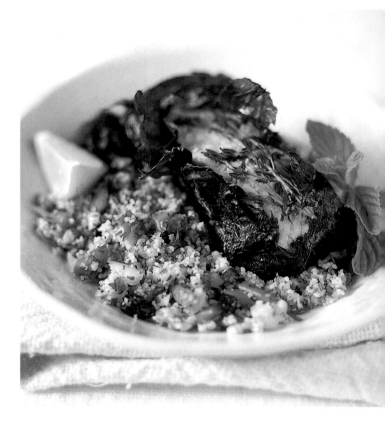

Pour boiling water over the salted vine leaves and leave for 5 minutes before rinsing well and squeezing to remove excess water.

Spread a vine leaf out on a board and place a salmon fillet on top. Season with salt and pepper and put a couple of thyme sprigs on top of the fish. Fold over the leaf and place another leaf on top, wrapping it underneath. Place two more leaves on top and wrap underneath. Lightly grease with olive oil on both sides. Make three more parcels in the same way.

Heat a griddle to medium high or preheat the oven to 400°F. Cook the fish parcels on both sides for 6–12 minutes depending on the thickness and heat of the griddle, or bake in the oven for 10–15 minutes. Press lightly to make sure the fish is firm. Leave to rest for a few minutes before serving; the fish can be served hot or cold.

Meanwhile, make the couscous: cook the fennel, beans, and garlic in the olive oil for about 20 minutes in a covered saucepan. Season with salt and pepper, stirring periodically and dropping any condensation from the lid inside to make the vegetables cook through. When the beans are just soft, add the raisins, ground fennel seeds, and cinnamon and mix. Add the couscous, mix briefly and then add ⅓ cup water. Stir well until the water has been absorbed by the couscous, then set aside for 5 minutes.

Mix the couscous well again to fluff it up. Stir in the chopped herbs and fennel fronds, if any, and serve hot or at room temperature with the salmon wrapped in vine leaves, and harissa and lemon wedges.

Fiber rating: MEDIUM

Per serving: 3.6g fiber, 385 Calories, 25g fat, 4g saturated fat, 1.12g sodium

Tuna niçoise with a pulse

To make this as an appetizer, you might want to increase the amount of fish a little. I have sometimes made this dish adding 5oz. unpeeled new potatoes to increase the fiber and carbohydrate content. **Serves 2 as a main dish or 4 as an appetizer or light lunch**

Scant cup (5oz.) cooked chickpeas

2 heaping tablespoons coarsely chopped or torn basil

2 tablespoons lemon juice

4 tablespoons extra virgin olive oil, plus extra for drizzling

Salt and freshly ground pepper

1 cup green beans

10 cherry tomatoes, cut in half

2 ounces arugula or other green salad leaf

11oz. fresh tuna steak

½ cup black olives or 4 heaping teaspoons tapenade

Lemon wedges, to serve

Mix the chickpeas with the basil, 1 tablespoon of the lemon juice and 2 tablespoons of the olive oil. Season with pepper, mix and leave to marinate.

Cook the green beans in boiling water for a few minutes until just tender, drain well and place in a large salad bowl. Add the tomatoes and arugula, season with salt and pepper and add the remaining lemon juice and olive oil, but don't mix until ready to serve or the arugula will become limp.

Heat a griddle pan or grill and drizzle a dash of oil on both sides of the tuna steak. Cook briefly, as tuna tastes delicious served raw in the middle like rare roast beef: allow about 1 minute each side, depending on how thick the tuna is. Remember that it will continue to cook after it is removed from the heat. Cook through if you prefer. Break the tuna in half if you want to see whether it's cooked—you can always serve two pieces arranged one above the other. Season with salt and pepper.

Add the chickpeas to the salad; mix and divide between serving plates. Place the tuna on top of the salad and serve with olives or a dollop of tapenade on top and a wedge of lemon to squeeze over.

Fiber rating: HIGH
Per serving (main dish): 7g fiber, 564 Calories, 35g fat, 6g saturated fat, 1.02g sodium

Scallop salad with olives, broccoli, and beans

Serve with toast or whole new potatoes to include some carbohydrates and fiber in the menu. You could increase the scallops if you wanted to make a more substantial dish. **Serves 4**

1 cup broccoli, cut into florets

1 cup green beans, topped and tailed

6oz. fava beans (picked weight), podded

1 red bell pepper, seeded and cut into small thin strips

16 good-quality black olives

4 tablespoons extra virgin olive oil, plus extra for drizzling

2 tablespoons lemon juice or vinegar

Salt and freshly ground black pepper

8 large scallops, total weight 12–14oz.

2 heaping tablespoons chopped fresh herbs, such as basil and parsley

Steam the broccoli and green beans until just cooked. Boil the fava beans in water until just cooked. Remove some of the pale outer skin from the fava beans if very large: the contrast in color works well. Place all the cooked vegetables in a bowl and add the red pepper, olives, olive oil, and lemon juice or vinegar. Season with salt and pepper and mix briefly.

Heat a griddle or skillet and drizzle a little oil over the scallops. Season with salt and pepper and cook briefly on both sides for about 2–4 minutes, depending on their size.

Mix the herbs with the vegetables and serve right away on one large or four individual plates with the scallops on top.

Fiber rating: HIGH
Per serving: 5.3g fiber, 271 Calories, 14g fat, 2g saturated fat, 0.55g sodium

Broiled polenta with shrimp, venetian style

If you don't like polenta (cornmeal), the shrimp are delicious with simply boiled potatoes or even pasta, but less authentic! Try to find good-quality polenta which is unrefined as opposed to instant and has a higher fiber content. **Serves 4**

1 cup polenta

Salt and freshly ground black pepper

3 tablespoons extra virgin olive oil, plus extra for the polenta

9oz. podded fava beans (fresh or frozen)

1½ cups podded peas (fresh or frozen)

1 small onion, chopped

1 large garlic clove, chopped

2 medium ripe tomatoes, diced

2 tablespoons dry white vermouth

2 heaping tablespoons basil, chopped or torn

3½ cups peeled large raw shrimp

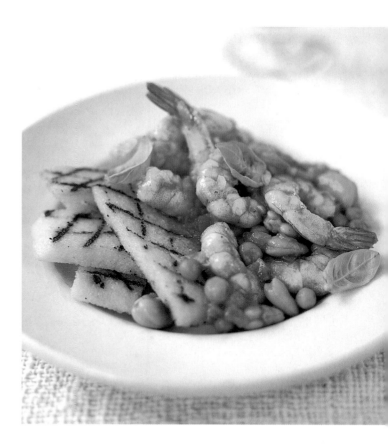

To make the polenta, bring 3 cups water to a boil with a good pinch of salt and slowly pour in the polenta. Mix with a whisk until it thickens, then stir periodically with a wooden spoon for 40 minutes over a gentle heat until cooked. Follow manufacturer's instructions if using instant. Pour onto a flat plate and leave to cool.

Just before serving, heat a griddle. Cut the polenta into strips or triangles and lightly smear the pieces with olive oil. (You might not need to use all the polenta.) Cook on a high heat on both sides until the polenta lifts off easily. Keep warm.

Cook the fava beans and peas separately in boiling water until tender. The pale outer skin of large fava beans can be quite tough, so remove it, revealing the darker inner bean. This will reduce the final quantity, so perhaps remove the skins for just half the beans or only the large ones. Set aside.

Cook the onion in 2 tablespoons of the olive oil for 5 minutes, until soft. Add the garlic and cooked fava beans and peas. Season with salt and pepper and mix briefly. Add the

diced tomatoes and cook until they reduce into a thick sauce. Add the vermouth and cook a minute more. Add the basil, then transfer to a bowl.

Rinse the pan, add the remaining olive oil and cook the shrimp on a medium–high heat for about 3–5 minutes on both sides, depending on their size, until golden brown. Add the bean mixture and mix briefly.

Place the broiled polenta on serving plates with the shrimp mixture and serve right away.

Fiber rating: HIGH
Per serving: 7g fiber, 383 Calories, 12g fat, 2g saturated fat, 0.8g sodium

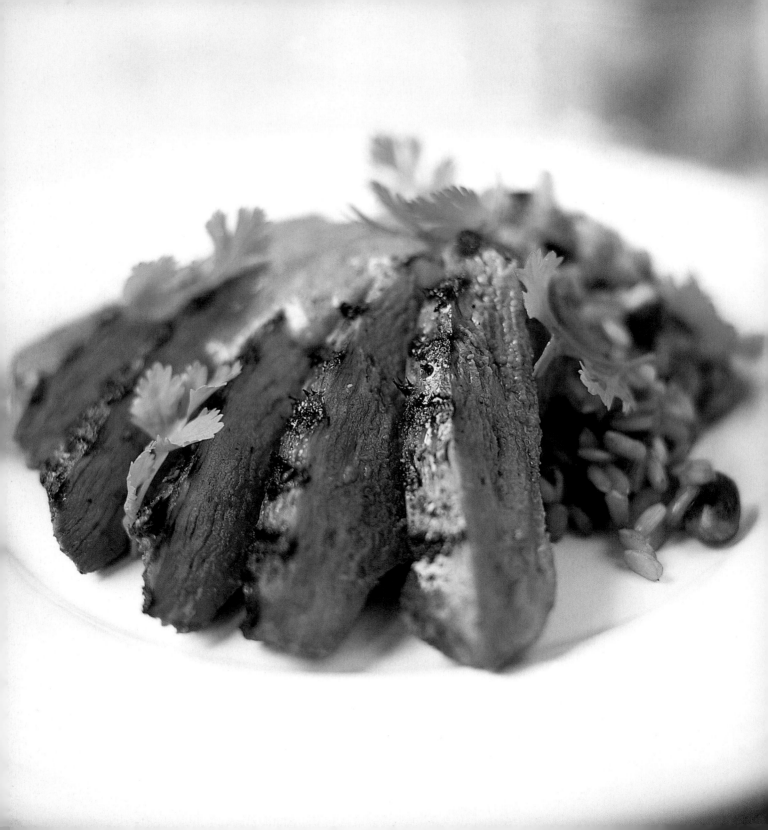

Meat

5

Venison stir-fry with zucchini and mushrooms

Zucchini and mushrooms are low-fiber vegetables, so if you need more high-fiber vegetables try snow peas and peppers. Venison is delicious and is a relatively low-fat meat, but beef or pork also work well. Serve with white or brown rice. **Serves 4**

14oz. lean venison haunch or fillet
1 medium carrot
5oz. shiitake, oyster, or chestnut mushrooms
1 smallish zucchini
2 tablespoons sunflower oil
½ teaspoon Chinese five spice (optional)

2 garlic cloves, sliced
1 heaping teaspoon finely grated or chopped fresh ginger root
2 tablespoons soy sauce
2 heaping tablespoons coarsely chopped cilantro

Prepare all the ingredients before cooking as stir-frying is a quick cooking process and you need all ingredients at hand. Cut the venison into thin strips. Peel the carrot then, still using the peeler, cut the carrot into long, thin strips. Cut the mushrooms into small or thin strips. Coarsely grate the zucchini.

Heat 1 tablespoon of the sunflower oil in a large wok over a high heat. Add the venison strips and the Chinese five spice, if using, and brown the meat quickly on both sides for about 1 minute. As soon as it is cooked, remove from the wok and set aside.

Heat the remaining sunflower oil and add the garlic and ginger root, cooking briefly. Add the carrot, mushrooms, and zucchini and cook for a further 2 minutes, stirring frequently. **When** the vegetables are just cooked, add the soy sauce, cilantro, and venison. Mix briefly and serve right away.

Fiber rating: LOW
Per serving: 0.7g fiber, 186 Calories, 8g fat, 2g saturated fat, 0.35g sodium

Garam masala duck breasts

A simple dish to prepare (see picture on page 96). Delicious with Saffron and Raisin Rice (see page 128) or a chickpea salad for extra fiber. Use ready-prepared garam masala if you wish, though home-made is far superior. **Serves 2 as a main dish or 4 as an appetizer**

½ cup (4½ oz.) low-fat plain yogurt
1 heaping teaspoon cornstarch
2 large skinless duck breasts, about 11oz. total weight
1 tablespoon coarsely chopped fresh cilantro, to serve

For the garam masala
1 teaspoon cardamom seeds (removed from pods)
1 small cinnamon stick, broken up
1 teaspoon cloves
1 teaspoon black peppercorns
2 teaspoons cumin seeds
2 teaspoons coriander seeds

To make the garam masala, grind all the ingredients in a spice grinder or mortar and pestle until fine. This can be prepared in advance. You will not need all of it for this recipe, but it keeps well in a sealed container for several months if all the ingredients are fresh when first prepared.

Put the yogurt, cornstarch, and 2 heaping teaspoons garam masala in a shallow bowl and mix well. Place the duck breasts in the bowl and turn to cover completely in the marinade. Cover the bowl and leave in the fridge for 4 hours or overnight (the flavor will improve if left overnight).

Remove the duck from the fridge 30 minutes before cooking. Heat a griddle to medium high or a grill to high. Remove most of the yogurt mixture from the duck and cook the breasts for about 8–10 minutes, turning over halfway through. Cook a little longer if you prefer your duck cooked through. Set aside to rest for 5 minutes before serving.

Place the yogurt mixture in a saucepan and gently bring to a boil. Cook briefly and add a dash of water if the mixture is too thick.

Serve the duck with the warm yogurt dressing on top and a scattering of cilantro for color.

Fiber rating: LOW
Per serving (main course): 0g fiber, 270 Calories, 11g fat, 3g saturated fat, 0.21g sodium

Quail stuffed with apricots and wild mushrooms

To make this dish with poussin instead of quail, allow one small poussin per person and increase the cooking time. Game and poultry work well with dried fruits and apricots are a good source of fiber. **Serves 4**

2 tablespoons olive oil
1 large red onion, finely chopped
1 large garlic clove, chopped
1 heaping tablespoon chopped sage
¾ oz. dried wild mushrooms such as porcini, soaked in just enough hot water to cover
½ cup dried apricots, chopped
3½ oz. cooked pearl barley
1 teaspoon grated or chopped fresh ginger root or stem ginger
Salt and freshly ground black pepper
8 quail or 4 small poussin
Green bean and arugula salad, to serve (optional)

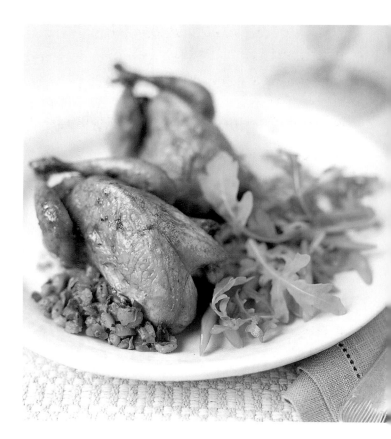

Heat the olive oil in a saucepan and gently cook the onion and garlic for about 10 minutes until soft and transparent, then add the sage.

Drain the mushrooms, reserving the soaking water, chop them and add to the onions along with the apricots. Cook for a minute, then add the mushroom water, discarding any sediment. Add the cooked pearl barley and ginger and simmer gently until all the mushroom liquid has evaporated. Season with salt and pepper. Set aside to cool. (Never stuff a bird with warm stuffing unless cooking it right away.) The stuffing can be prepared in advance and stored in the fridge, but remove it from the fridge 15 minutes before using.

Place a small roasting pan in the oven and preheat to 400°F. Stuff the quail with the mushroom mixture. Tie the legs together to keep the stuffing from falling out, place breast up on the roasting tray and season with salt and pepper.

Roast the birds for 10 minutes. Turn them over and place back in the oven for a further 10–15 minutes. Turn the heat down to 350°F, turn the birds breast up again and cook for a further 5–10 minutes. Add a dash of water at this stage to prevent the juices from evaporating. Remove from the oven and leave to rest for 10 minutes before eating.

Cut the quail in half lengthwise, pour the cooking juices on top and serve with a green bean and arugula salad. If there is any stuffing not used, it can be reheated at the last minute and served alongside.

Fiber rating LOW
Per serving, not including green bean and arugula salad: 1.3g fiber, 424 Calories, 26g fat, 6g saturated fat, 0.59g sodium

Pot-roasted beef brisket

This can be used as the basis for various dishes including Beef and Potato Hash on page 48, in which case the extra can be enjoyed another day for a main course with mustard and simply roasted vegetables. Plain rather than salted brisket is used for a subtler flavor. **Serves 6–8**

3lbs. 5oz. beef brisket, unrolled
¾ cup red wine
1 teaspoon black peppercorns
1 tablespoon sea salt

2 small star anise or 1 level teaspoon Chinese five spice (optional)
2 large carrots, halved
1 large onion, quartered
4 garlic cloves

Preheat the oven to 350°F. Place the beef in a casserole or high-sided roasting pan.

Pour over the wine, peppercorns, salt, and star anise, if using. Scatter over the vegetables and just enough hot water to submerge the beef slightly. (You want to half-steam the meat, not boil it or dry it out.)

Cover with a lid or aluminum foil and cook in the oven for about 3 hours. The beef should be soft and tender and flake easily. Once it is cooked, leave to rest for 30 minutes.

Fiber rating: LOW
Per serving (6 people): 0.9g fiber, 596 Calories, 28g fat, 11g saturated fat, 0.94g sodium

Persian chicken with rice

This is a form of pilaf or pilaw—a Middle Eastern method of cooking rice, which involves coating it in oil and spices before cooking it in stock. This dish goes well with a simple cucumber and yogurt salad and can be served as part of a southern Mediterranean buffet. **Serves 4**

4 tablespoons extra virgin olive oil
1 medium onion, finely chopped
1 cup cashew nuts
4 x chicken thighs, skinned, boned, and cut into small cubes (or use chicken breasts for a lower fat version)
1 heaping teaspoon cumin seeds, lightly crushed
2 garlic cloves, finely chopped

Salt and freshly ground black pepper
½ cup dried cranberries
6 cardamom pods
1 cinnamon stick
1¼ cups brown basmati rice
1 teaspoon ground allspice
Large pinch of saffron, soaked in 2 tablespoons water or chicken stock
2 cups chicken stock or water
2 tablespoons chopped cilantro

Heat the olive oil in a large saucepan or deep skillet, add the onion and cashew nuts and cook on a medium heat until the onion is soft and the nuts have infused in the oil. Increase the heat a little, add the chicken pieces and cumin seeds and cook for about 5 minutes until the chicken is lightly browned, stirring occasionally so all sides are cooked. Add the garlic at this point to prevent it from burning, season with salt and pepper and stir briefly for 1 minute.

Add the cranberries, cardamom, cinnamon stick, rice, allspice, and saffron and briefly mix all the ingredients together. Then add the chicken stock, giving a final stir, cover with a lid and cook the mixture at a gentle simmer for about 10–15 minutes until the rice is cooked and the liquid has evaporated.

Serve with the chopped cilantro scattered on top. Remember that the cardamom and cinnamon are left whole to infuse their flavor into the dish and should not be eaten: you might want to remind your guests of this before serving!

Fiber rating: MEDIUM
Per serving: 3.1g fiber, 576 Calories, 27g fat, 5g saturated fat, 0.65g sodium

Meatballs with chickpeas

These are often called kofta meatballs and are traditional Morocco fare. I have included chickpeas in the recipe, but other pulses such as borlotti or flageolet beans can be substituted. Serving with wholewheat pita bread will increase the fiber. **Serves 4**

1 heaping teaspoon cumin seeds

1 heaping teaspoon coriander seeds

1 large garlic clove, crushed with salt

18oz. lean ground beef

2 heaping tablespoons fresh wholewheat breadcrumbs

1 medium egg, beaten (optional)

1 tablespoon coarsely chopped fresh cilantro

Salt and freshly ground black pepper

2 tablespoons olive oil

14-oz. can cooked chickpeas, drained and rinsed

14-oz. can chopped tomatoes

For serving (optional)

Low-fat live yogurt, coarsely chopped fresh cilantro and warm pita bread

Dry-roast the cumin and coriander seeds in a small skillet or saucepan until light golden brown—watch carefully as they can burn very easily. Remove and grind using a mortar and pestle or spice grinder. (You can use ready-ground spices but the smoky aroma is lost.) Add the spices and puréed garlic to the ground meat and mix with the breadcrumbs, egg, if using, cilantro, salt and pepper. Mix well and roll into 24 small balls about the size of a walnut.

Heat the oil in a large sauté pan or skillet and cook the meatballs on a medium heat, turning frequently, until colored all over. Cook in batches if need be. Drain any fat from the pan with a spoon and discard.

Add the chickpeas to the meatballs. Mix briefly, reduce the heat and cook for a few minutes. Add the tomatoes and simmer gently until all the liquid is reduced, making a sweet-flavored sauce. Leave to rest for at least 10 minutes off the heat, then add a dash of water to loosen slightly, while still leaving a thick sauce. Reheat briefly at this stage if necessary.

Serve with a dollop of yogurt and a sprinkling of cilantro; warm pita or wholewheat bread is good for mopping up the juices.

Fiber rating: MEDIUM

Per serving, including egg, not including serving suggestion: 3.6g fiber, 353 Calories, 19g fat, 6g saturated fat, 0.62g sodium

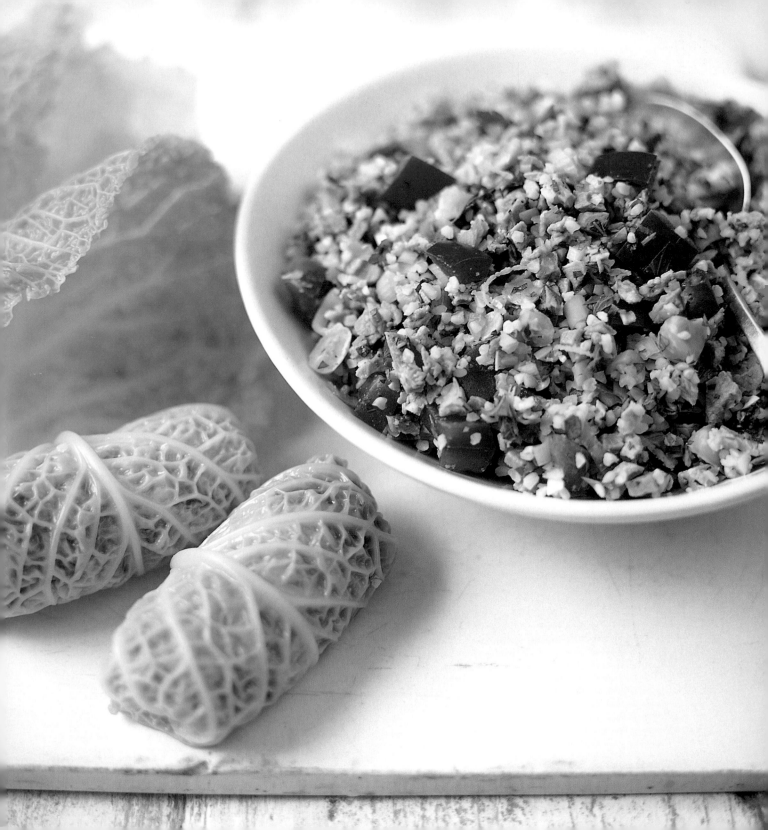

Middle Eastern lamb wrapped in cabbage leaves

I always love recipes that use up leftovers and this is much more glamorous than shepherd's pie! Sumac is a spice that can be easily found in any Middle Eastern grocery store. **Serves** 4

9-oz. cooked leg of lamb, trimmed of any fat
⅓ cup bulgur wheat
½ cup pine nuts or hazelnuts, roasted in a medium oven for 10 minutes and coarsely chopped
2oz. scallions, finely chopped
2 heaping tablespoons coarsely chopped flat-leaf parsley
2 heaping tablespoons coarsely chopped mint
1 red bell pepper, seeded and diced
Juice of 2 large lemons (10 tablespoons)
1 tablespoon sumac (or grated lemon zest if unavailable)
Salt and freshly ground black pepper
About 16–20 cabbage leaves

If you have a grinder, grind the lamb on a coarse setting; otherwise finely chop it. Don't be tempted to use a food processor, because this will result in a purée.

Soak the bulgur wheat in enough boiling water just to cover. Leave for 10 minutes until it softens, drain in a colander for a few minutes if the water has not all been soaked up, and press briefly to remove any excess water.

Place the ground lamb in a bowl and add the bulgur wheat, nuts, scallions, parsley, mint, red pepper, lemon juice, sumac or lemon zest, salt and pepper. Taste for seasoning and leave to infuse. This can be prepared in advance.

Bring a large saucepan of water to a boil. Add the cabbage leaves and blanch them for about 5 minutes until just soft. Refresh them in cold water and leave to drain well.

This dish can be served as ready-made rolls, or you can serve separately and let people wrap the lamb themselves. Place a spoonful of the lamb mixture in the middle of each leaf and wrap up. Try to get the right proportion of lamb to cabbage, so the cabbage does not overpower the meat.

Fiber rating: MEDIUM
Per serving: 4.7g fiber, 319 Calories, 15g fat, 3g saturated fat, 0.36g sodium

Mediterranean chicken and prune

stew *Prunes have a reputation for being too wholesome but their sweet, rich flavor is perfect for any meat stew and gives color to the sauce as well. Serve with Wholesome Mashed Tatties (page 118) and steamed green vegetables for extra fiber.* **Serves 4**

4 large chicken thighs, skinned and boned, about 13oz. total weight

2 tablespoons extra virgin olive oil

4 strips pancetta or smoked bacon, diced

1 medium onion, quartered and sliced

4 medium carrots, cut in half lengthwise and sliced at an angle

Salt and freshly ground black pepper

2 garlic cloves, sliced

1 heaping tablespoon chopped thyme or rosemary

1 cup pitted prunes

1 heaping teaspoon cornstarch, mixed with 1 tablespoon water

1⅓ cups chicken stock

Cut the chicken thighs into large cubes. Pour the olive oil into a large sauté pan or flameproof casserole and cook the chicken on a medium-high heat until golden brown on all sides. Remove from the pan, leaving any oil behind, and set aside.

Add the pancetta or bacon to the pan and brown lightly. Add the onion and carrots and cook gently for 10 minutes, stirring periodically. Season with salt and pepper and add the garlic and herb. Stir and cook for a minute more.

Return the chicken and add the prunes, mix briefly and add the cornstarch paste and chicken stock. Bring to a simmer, cover with a lid and cook gently for 20 minutes.

Fiber rating: MEDIUM

Per serving: 3.6g fiber, 347 Calories, 16g fat, 4g saturated fat, 0.69g sodium

Beef and lima bean stew with

peppers *Other pulses such as cannellini beans can be substituted for the lima beans. Always wash beans well to drain them of the cooking water which causes most of the flatulence associated with beans and pulses.* **Serves 4**

2 tablespoons extra virgin olive oil

13oz. lean stewing beef, cubed

1 medium onion, chopped

1 medium carrot, chopped (unpeeled)

1 celery stick, chopped

2 small red or green bell peppers, seeded and cut into chunks

2 garlic cloves, chopped

2¼–2½ cups lima beans, rinsed and drained

Salt and freshly ground black pepper

⅓ cup sherry vinegar or red wine vinegar

1 heaping teaspoon cornstarch

1¾ cups beef stock or water

Warm crusty bread, for serving (optional)

Preheat the oven to 300°F.

Pour the olive oil into a flameproof casserole and heat to medium high. Seal the beef in the oil, turning once, until golden brown. Remove from the casserole and set aside.

Add the onion, carrot, celery, peppers, and garlic to the casserole and cook gently for 10 minutes, stirring occasionally. Add the lima beans and beef, mix briefly, then season with salt and pepper. Mix the cornstarch with the vinegar and stock or water and add to casserole. Stir, then cover with a lid and place in the oven. Cook for about 1½–2 hours, until the beef is tender.

Serve with warm crusty bread, either wholewheat or white, depending on your fiber requirements.

Fiber rating: HIGH

Per serving, not including bread: 5g fiber, 259 Calories, 10g fat, 2g saturated fat, 1.07g sodium

Broiled chicken sandwich on pumpernickel bread with roast peppers and hummus

Pumpernickel bread is made from very coarse meal rye flour. It is also a very high-fiber bread, so a little can go a long way! **Serves 2**

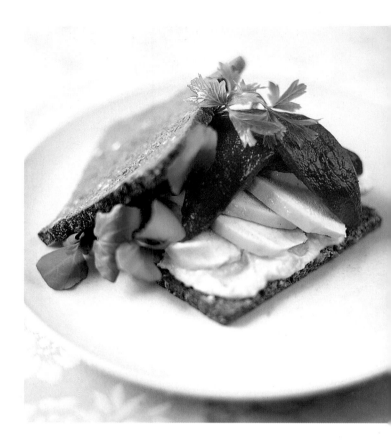

5oz. chicken breast

1 red bell pepper

4 slices pumpernickel bread (check the fiber table on page 24 if you need to use a lower fiber bread)

2 heaping tablespoons hummus

Salt and freshly ground black pepper

2 dill or flat-leaf parsley sprigs (optional)

2 large watercress sprigs

Preheat the grill to medium-high and broil the chicken breast for about 10 minutes, depending on the thickness. When it is cooked through, set aside to rest.

Broil the pepper, place in a plastic bag to loosen the skin, then remove the skin, halve the pepper and remove the seeds.

Lightly toast the pumpernickel bread on both sides, being careful not to break it as it's quite fragile. Place a piece on each serving plate. Smear the bread with hummus. Thinly slice the chicken breast and divide between the slices of bread. Lay a red pepper half over the chicken. Season with salt and pepper, then place a sprig of dill or parsley, if using, and some watercress on top.

Cover with the remaining pumpernickel and serve right away. Cut in half with a sharp serrated knife for best results.

Fiber rating: HIGH

Per serving: 7.2g fiber, 359 Calories, 10g fat, 1g saturated fat, 0.73g sodium

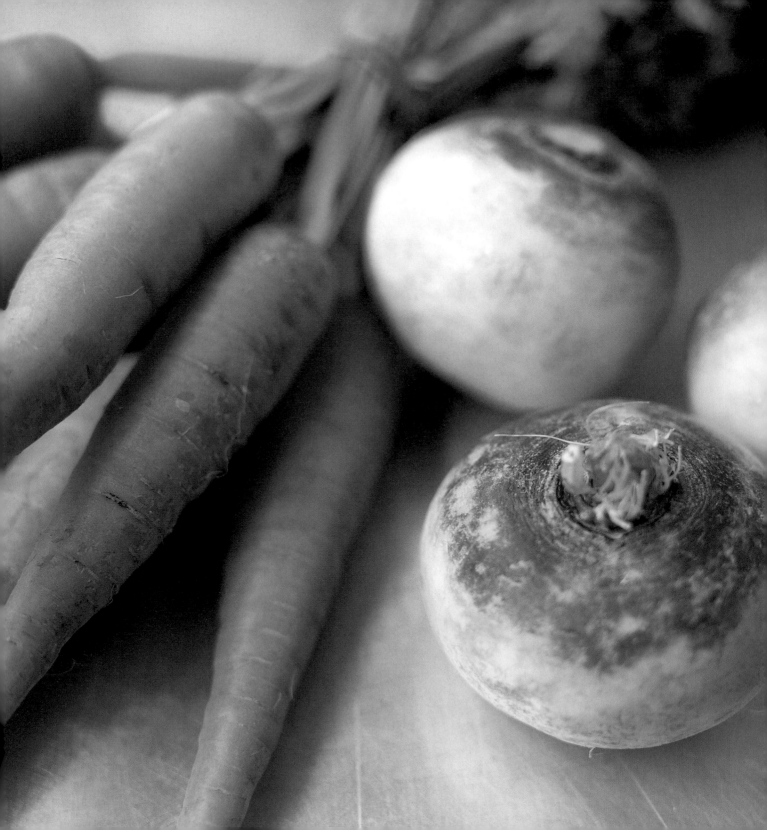

6

Vegetables and Tofu

Stir-fried asparagus with sesame seeds

A quick and easy recipe to use when asparagus is in season and you are bored of eating it just boiled with olive oil or butter. It can be made more elaborate by adding ginger or other vegetables. Serve with stir-fried noodles or steamed rice. **Serves 2**

8–10 (7oz.) trimmed asparagus spears
1 tablespoon sunflower oil
1 heaping tablespoon sesame seeds
1 garlic clove, thinly sliced
1 tablespoon oyster sauce
1 tablespoon soy sauce

Cut the asparagus at an angle into thin strips, so that it is easier to cook in a wok.

Heat the oil in a wok and add the asparagus and sesame seeds. Stir and cook for 2 minutes. Add the garlic and cook for 1 further minute.

Add the oyster sauce and soy sauce, stirring so that asparagus briefly steams in the liquid. Place on plates and serve right away at room temperature.

Fiber rating: LOW
Per serving: 2.2g fiber, 120 Calories, 10g fat, 1g saturated fat, 0.67g sodium

Asparagus and red onion tart

If asparagus is not in season, substitute broiled red bell peppers. If only fat asparagus is available, cut in half lengthwise. Use wholewheat pastry if you wish to increase the fiber content.

Serves 4 as a main dish or 6 as an appetizer

9oz. shortcrust pastry
4 medium red onions, quartered and finely sliced
2 garlic cloves, thinly sliced
1 heaping tablespoon chopped thyme
2 tablespoons olive oil
2 tablespoons balsamic vinegar
12–16 trimmed thin asparagus
²/₃ cup ricotta cheese
Salt and freshly ground black pepper

Roll out the pastry to ⅛-inch thickness and use to line a 9½-inch metal tart pan. Press the pastry gently into the tin, trimming the edge, but making sure that it comes a little above the side of the pan, so that when it cooks it doesn't shrink too much. Leave to rest in the fridge for about 15 minutes.

Preheat the oven to 350°F.

Gently cook the onions, garlic, and thyme in the olive oil for about 20 minutes until soft and lightly caramelized, stirring periodically. Add the balsamic vinegar and cook until it has completely reduced into the onions. Set aside.

Cook the asparagus in salted boiling water for about 3 minutes, until just tender. Refresh in cold water and dry on kitchen paper towels.

Prick the pastry base with a fork and bake for about 15 minutes. Once the pastry is a light golden brown and completely cooked remove from the oven. Increase the oven to 400°F. Place the onion mixture in the pastry case, spreading it out evenly. Trim the asparagus to fit like wheel spokes on top of the onion mixture, place in position and dollop the ricotta all over. Season with salt and pepper and put back in the oven for another 5–10 minutes to brown the ricotta lightly. Be careful not to burn the edges of the pastry—turn the heat down a little if your oven is fierce. Serve warm.

Fiber rating: LOW
Per serving (appetizer): 2.7g fiber, 294 Calories, 18g fat, 6g saturated fat, 0.38g sodium

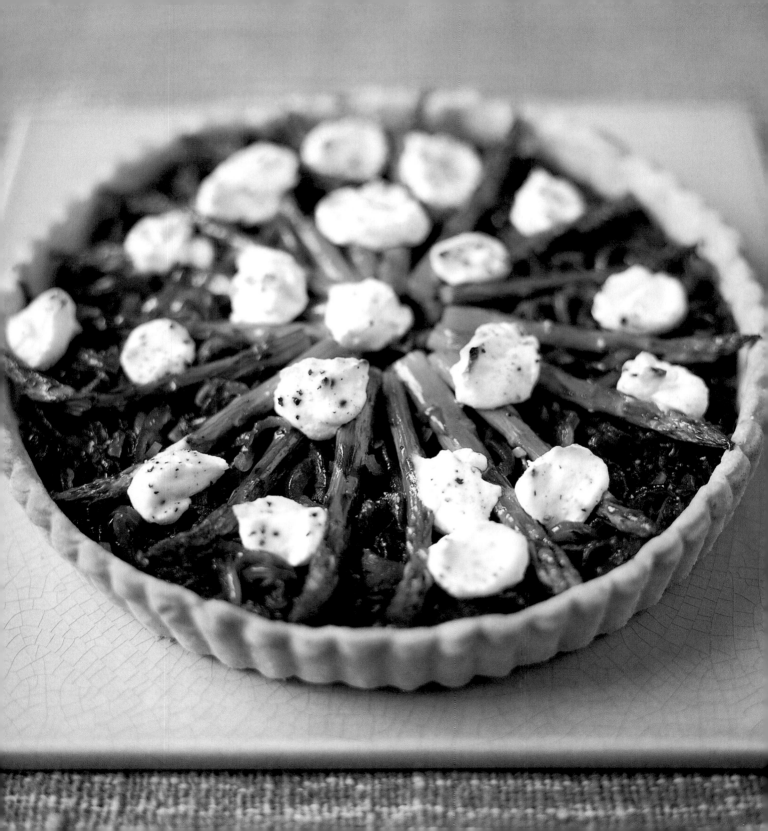

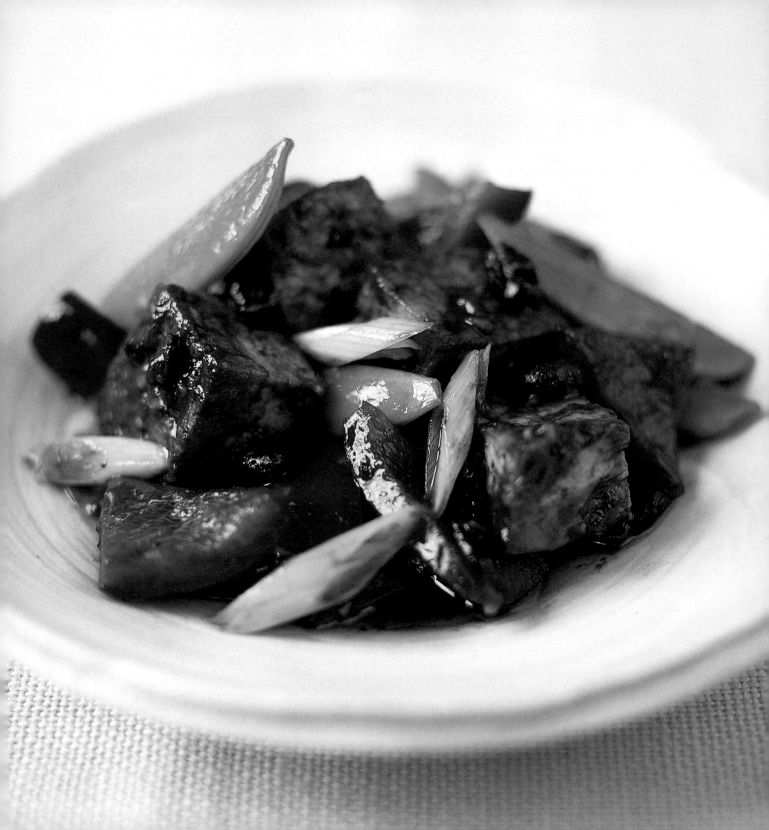

Stir-fried tofu with peppers and black bean sauce

Good Asian food stores sell fermented black beans which make for a more authentic sauce. If not, black bean sauce is more easily available, being stocked by most big supermarkets. Serve with steamed white rice. **Serves 4**

- 10½ oz. tofu, drained on kitchen towels for 10 minutes
- 2 tablespoons sunflower oil
- 2 large red bell peppers, seeded and cut into triangular shapes
- 2 handfuls snow peas or sugar snap peas
- 3 large scallions, sliced
- 2 garlic cloves, chopped or grated
- 2 heaping teaspoons fresh chopped or grated ginger
- 1 tablespoon hoisin sauce
- 1 heaping tablespoon black bean sauce or fermented black beans
- 1 teaspoon chile paste (optional)
- 4 tablespoons Chinese wine or sake, sherry or water

After preparing the vegetables, cut the tofu into 1-inch cubes. **Heat** the sunflower oil in a large wok and cook the tofu on a medium-high heat until golden brown on all sides. Set aside to drain on paper towels.

Add the peppers, peas, and scallions to the wok and cook for 2 minutes, stirring frequently. Add the garlic and ginger root and cook for 1 further minute.

Finally add the hoisin sauce, black bean sauce or fermented black beans, chile paste, if using, Chinese wine or alternative and 3 tablespoons water. Cook briefly, then add the tofu, turning the heat down to low. Mix all the ingredients together, cooking the sauce further until thick, and serve.

Fiber rating: LOW
Per serving: 2.6g fiber, 170 Calories, 9g fat, 1g saturated fat, 0.21g sodium

Tofu curry with pumpkin and broccoli

If lime leaves are hard to find, you can substitute lemon grass. Both have a fragrant acidity to counteract the richness of the coconut milk. Substitute carrots for the pumpkin to increase the fiber content of the dish. **Serves 4**

- 10½ oz. tofu (beancurd), drained on kitchen towels for 10 minutes
- 2 tablespoons sunflower oil
- 8oz. pumpkin (peeled weight), cut into 1-inch cubes
- 1 cup broccoli, cut into small pieces, including the stems
- 1 heaping teaspoon coriander seeds
- 1 heaping teaspoon cumin seeds
- 14-oz. can coconut milk
- 1 medium tomato, diced
- ½–1 teaspoon red curry paste
- 2 tablespoons Thai fish sauce
- 3 lime leaves or 2 medium lemon grass sticks, cut into chunks
- 1–1½ cups baby spinach leaves
- 1 tablespoon lime juice
- 2 heaping tablespoons coarsely chopped Thai basil or cilantro
- Steamed jasmine rice, to serve (optional)

Cut the tofu into 1-inch cubes.

Heat the sunflower oil in a large wok and fry the tofu on a medium-high heat until golden brown on all sides. Set aside to drain on kitchen paper towels.

Add the pumpkin and broccoli to the wok with the coriander and cumin seeds. Cook for a minute to seal the vegetables in the oil and lightly roast the spices. Add the coconut milk, tomato, red curry paste, fish sauce, and lime leaves or lemon grass. Mix well and simmer gently for 15 minutes until the vegetables are just tender.

Add the tofu, spinach, lime juice, and basil or cilantro. Mix well, cooking the spinach until just wilted, then serve right away with steamed jasmine rice.

Fiber rating: LOW
Per serving not including rice: 2.4g fiber, 164 Calories, 10g fat, 1g saturated fat, 0.76g sodium

Asian steamed tofu with mushrooms and greens

Several tofu recipes have been included in this book as it is a lean source of protein, rich in calcium. But it has little fiber so is best when you need low fiber in your diet. **Serves 4 as an appetizer or light meal**

10½ oz. tofu (beancurd), drained on kitchen towels for 10 minutes	**For the marinade**
2 tablespoons sunflower oil	1 heaping teaspoon finely grated fresh ginger root
7oz. fresh shiitake or straw mushrooms	1 garlic clove, finely chopped or grated
1 garlic clove, sliced	1 heaping teaspoon miso paste
11oz. mustard greens	2 tablespoons soy sauce
Steamed rice, to serve (optional)	2 tablespoons sake, sherry or dry vermouth

To make the marinade, mix all the ingredients together in a bowl.

Cut the tofu into 1-inch cubes and add to the marinade, carefully coating the tofu without breaking it. Leave for a couple of hours in the fridge.

Remove the tofu from the marinade and steam for 5 minutes, then set aside in the steamer to keep warm.

Heat the sunflower oil in a large wok and cook the mushrooms with the garlic until soft. Add the broccoli or greens and a dash of the water from the steamed tofu and cook gently with a lid on (or covered with aluminum foil) for 15 minutes, stirring periodically. When the greens are just tender, place these and the mushrooms on a warmed plate.

Put the marinade ingredients into the wok, cook briefly, then add a dash of the tofu steaming water to loosen the sauce if need be. Set aside.

Place the tofu on top of the mushrooms and greens and drizzle the hot sauce on top.

Serve right away with steamed rice.

Fiber rating: LOW
Per serving not including rice: 1.8g fiber, 160 Calories, 9g fat, 1g saturated fat, 0.1g sodium

Thai noodles with tofu and vegetables

Traditionally this recipe requires preserved turnip, found in any good Thai food shop, though it is not essential. Include 1 heaping tablespoon of it when adding the vegetables, if you wish. **Serves 4**

9oz. tofu (beancurd), drained on kitchen towels for 10 minutes	2 garlic cloves, chopped
2½ cups rice noodles	1 teaspoon chile paste (optional)
2 tablespoons sunflower oil	1 tablespoon tamarind paste (or juice of 1 large lime)
2 eggs	3 tablespoons Thai fish sauce
2 yellow bell peppers, cut into triangular shapes	2 tablespoons salted peanuts, coarsely chopped
3 large scallions, sliced	2 heaping tablespoons coarsely chopped cilantro or Thai basil
1 heaping tablespoon preserved turnip (optional)	

Cut the tofu into 1-inch cubes.

Place the noodles in a large bowl or saucepan and pour boiling water over them. Leave for about 3–5 minutes until they loosen up and are al dente. Stir them around in the water to prevent them sticking together. Drain, refresh in cold water and drain again, leaving a little water to stop them sticking.

Have all the prepared vegetables and other ingredients on hand before you start as the rest of the dish will be cooked quickly.

Heat the sunflower oil in a large wok on a medium-high heat and add the cubed tofu, lightly browning on all sides for a few minutes. Remove and leave to drain on paper towels.

Break the eggs into the pan, breaking the yolks. Cook, folding the eggs slightly to break them into large pieces, rather than scrambling them. Push the eggs to the side and add the peppers, scallions, preserved turnip, garlic, and chile paste, if using, and cook, stirring periodically, for 3 minutes until the peppers are just tender. Add the tamarind paste and fish sauce, stir briefly, then add the tofu, noodles, and peanuts, mixing well. Finally add cilantro or basil and serve right away.

Fiber rating: LOW
Per serving: 1.9g fiber, 385 Calories, 15g fat, 2g saturated fat, 0.96g sodium

Potato-base pizza with zucchini, olives, and ricotta

A tasty wheat-free alternative to regular pizza. As with any pizza, the toppings can be adapted, they just should need very little time to cook, or be cooked already.

Serves 2 as a main dish or 4 as an appetizer

2 tablespoons olive oil, plus extra for greasing
1 large baking potato
Salt and freshly ground black pepper
1 large zucchini

½ cup ricotta cheese
2oz. tapenade or 12 large black pitted olives
1 heaping tablespoon chopped basil or thyme
Salad, to serve

Place a large baking sheet in the oven and preheat to 400°F. Cut a sheet of aluminum foil about 14 x 16 inches and smear with a little olive oil leaving an unoiled border of about 2 inches around the edge.

Peel and thinly slice the potato and arrange on the foil in a rectangular shape, overlapping slightly. Season with salt and pepper and drizzle 1 tablespoon of the oil on top.

Thinly slice the zucchini and scatter over, leaving a little gap around the edges as you would on a pizza base. Dollop the ricotta evenly across the top and scatter over the tapenade or olives. If using thyme, sprinkle it on the pizza now (basil should be added after cooking). Finally drizzle over the remaining oil and season with salt and pepper.

Remove the heated baking sheet from the oven and carefully place the foil holding the pizza on top. Cook in the oven for about 15–20 minutes until the edges are golden brown and the center soft and cooked.

Remove from the oven and, if using basil, scatter over the pizza now. Allow to rest for 5 minutes.

Cut into quarters and serve with salad.

Fiber rating: MEDIUM
Per serving (main course): 3.4g fiber, 317 Calories, 19g fat, 5g saturated fat, 1.05g sodium

Leek and yellow pepper bake

Lovely with simply broiled or roasted meat or fish. The latter makes for a particularly easy recipe as the whole meal comes from the oven and needs little assistance. It would also work well with Stuffed Quail (page 99) or Monkfish Kebabs (page 86). **Serves 4**

2 large yellow bell peppers
4 medium leeks (12oz.)
2 large garlic cloves, quartered
1 tablespoon chopped thyme

3 tablespoons extra virgin olive oil
Salt and freshly ground black pepper

Preheat the oven to 350°F.

Cut the peppers in half and discard the stem and seeds. Cut into large wedges.

Cut the leeks in half and then cut into 3-inch lengths.

Place the vegetables in a large gratin dish and mix with the garlic, thyme, oil, salt and pepper.

Cover with aluminum foil and bake in the oven for 20 minutes. Remove the foil and cook for a further 20 minutes, until the vegetables are soft. Serve.

Fiber rating: MEDIUM
Per serving: 4.1g fiber, 128 Calories, 9g fat, 1g saturated fat, 0.3g sodium

Mini pea and potato pasties

The peas can be substituted with other vegetables such as zucchini if you prefer. They should be cooked at the same time as the potatoes. The potatoes can also be peeled if a lower fiber option is needed.

Makes 12 pasties; serves 4–6

18oz. wholewheat or plain shortcrust pastry

1 medium onion, finely chopped

1 large garlic clove, finely chopped

2 tablespoons extra virgin olive oil

2 medium non-waxy potatoes, such as Idaho

Salt and freshly ground black pepper

1 cup frozen peas

1 heaping tablespoon coarsely chopped fresh mint

2 tablespoons water or milk, to glaze

Roll out the pastry to about ⅛ inches thick and 13 inches in diameter. Leave to rest in the fridge on a floured plate, folded if necessary, for about 15 minutes.

Cook the onion and garlic in the olive oil for a few minutes. Cut the potatoes into small dice and add to the onion. Season with salt and pepper and cover with a lid. Gently cook the potatoes, stirring frequently, for about 20 minutes until they are soft. Add the frozen peas and mint and cook for a further 5 minutes. Set aside to cool.

Preheat the oven to 400°F.

Take the pastry from the fridge and cut it into 12 discs of about 4-inch diameter, rerolling as necessary to use all the trimmings. Rest the pastry again if you have time as this helps prevent cracking and shrinkage when cooking.

To fill the pastry, brush the edge of pastry circles with a little water or milk and place about ½ tablespoon of the pea mixture in the center of each one. Fold up two sides of the pastry and pinch in the middle to seal, then fold up one other side, creating two seams and press the pastry together. Repeat on the other side so you have a square shape with four sealed lines. Alternatively fold over the pastry and seal down one side to make a half-moon shape.

Place the pasties on a baking sheet and brush with a little more water or milk to glaze. Cook in the oven for about 20 minutes until the pastry is cooked and golden brown.

Serve after resting for about 10 minutes. Don't worry if the parcels break their seal—they are just as tasty!

Fiber rating: MEDIUM
Per pasty, with wholewheat pastry: 3.2g fiber, 221 Calories, 14g fat, 4g saturated fat, 0.25g sodium

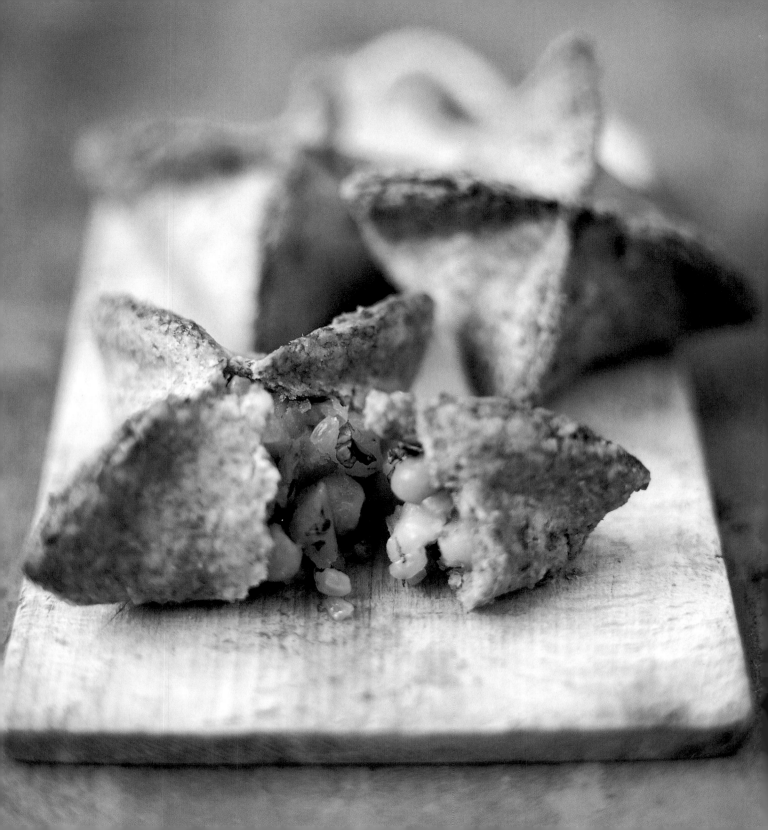

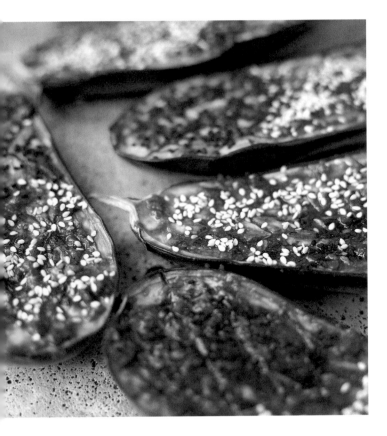

Broiled eggplant with miso

This recipe is very simple. Miso has a wonderful intense taste that is rich, salty, and tart. It is a base note to many Japanese recipes and keeps for ages in the fridge once opened. Traditionally red miso is used, but any good miso will work. **Serves 4 as a side dish or appetizer**

1¾ lbs. eggplant
Sea salt
2 level tablespoons miso

2 tablespoons mirin or sake, sherry or vermouth
2 teaspoons sugar
Black and white sesame seeds

Cut the eggplant in half lengthwise and score the cut sides in a criss-cross pattern, avoiding cutting too deep into the flesh and losing the shape. Sprinkle with salt and leave to sweat for 10 minutes. Rinse in water and squeeze dry, then wrap in kitchen paper towels.

Preheat the grill or oven to medium.

Broil or bake the eggplant for about 15 minutes until completely cooked. Some vegetables can be al dente but not eggplant.

Make the miso paste by mixing the miso with the mirin or alternative alcohol and the sugar. When the eggplant is cooked, smear the miso mixture over the top, so that it is completely covered. Sprinkle with the sesame seeds, covering half with white and the other half with black.

Serve warm, and with plain rice if serving as a light vegetarian main dish.

Fiber rating: MEDIUM
Per serving: 4.2g fiber, 92 Calories, 3g fat, 0g saturated fat, 0.76g sodium

Tofu-sesame dipping sauce with steamed vegetables

This is a tasty dipping sauce to eat with raw or steamed vegetables and is a different way of using tofu. Serve with boiled rice and a broiled piece of chicken for a complete meal. **Serves 4**

10½ oz. soft tofu (beancurd), drained on kitchen towels for 10 minutes

5 tablespoons sesame seeds

2 tablespoons rice wine vinegar

2 tablespoons soy sauce

For serving

1 cup broccoli, cut into thin florets

1 cup green beans

3 medium carrots, cut into strips

1 red bell pepper, seeded and sliced

Boiled rice (optional)

Place the tofu in a steamer. Bring to a boil, cover with a lid and cook for 10 minutes. A colander over a saucepan of boiling water works just as well if covered.

Toast the sesame seeds in a medium oven or on top of the stove in a skillet until golden brown. Reserve 1 heaping teaspoon for the garnish and grind the rest in a spice grinder or using a mortar and pestle.

Place the tofu, ground sesame seeds, vinegar, and soy sauce in a blender or food processor and blend until smooth. Pour into a serving bowl, and sprinkle with the reserved toasted sesame seeds just before serving.

Serve the vegetables steamed or raw, accompanied by the tofu dressing as a dipping sauce.

Fiber rating: MEDIUM

Per serving not including rice: 4.6g fiber, 174 Calories, 11g fat, 2g saturated fat, 0.14g sodium

Braised fennel with carrots

A simple combination of vegetables that tastes delicious with broiled fish or chicken. Zucchini can be substituted for carrots. Leave the carrots unpeeled to increase the fiber content of the dish and choose organic carrots that have no chemicals sprayed on the skin. **Serves 4**

14-oz. bulb fennel

4 medium carrots

3 tablespoons extra virgin olive oil

1 large garlic clove, chopped

Salt and freshly ground black pepper

1 heaping tablespoon chopped basil

Remove any fennel fronds, chop and set aside. Cut the fennel in half lengthways and slice into thin wedges. Cut the carrots in half lengthways and thinly slice at an angle.

Heat the oil in a large sauté pan and add the vegetables and garlic. Season with salt and pepper and cook on a medium-high heat, stirring periodically, for 20 minutes, so the vegetables just catch and brown lightly. Place a lid on the pan, reduce the heat and cook for a further 10–15 minutes, until the vegetables are tender. When lifting the lid to stir, add any condensation from the lid to moisten the vegetables and help them cook further.

When the vegetables are soft, add the basil and the reserved chopped fennel fronds and serve. This dish can be prepared in advance as it reheats well.

Fiber rating: MEDIUM

Per serving: 4.2g fiber, 97 Calories, 8g fat, 1g saturated fat, 0.48g sodium

Wholesome mashed tatties in their skins

A friend prepared mashed potatoes this way for me once, I suspect because she couldn't be bothered to peel all the potatoes. Since I realized that most of a potato's nutrients are just under the skin, I have always made mash at home like this. **Serves 4**

5 medium unpeeled potatoes (18oz.), any non-waxy variety that is good for mashing

Salt and freshly ground black pepper
½ stick unsalted butter
2 tablespoons milk
Good pinch of grated nutmeg

Cut the potatoes into large chunks—they should not be too small or the mash will become waterlogged.

Cook gently in salted boiling water for about 20 minutes until soft. Drain well and return back to the pan. Add the butter in small pieces and pour in the milk. Season with salt, pepper, and nutmeg. Mash to a purée and serve. Delicious with a variety of main courses from this book, such as Mediterranean Chicken and Prune Stew (see page 104).

Variation

For a lower fat recipe, use 5 tablespoons olive oil instead of milk and butter.

Fiber rating: MEDIUM
Per serving: 3.4g fiber, 315 Calories, 11g fat, 7g saturated fat, 0.26g sodium

Braised red cabbage with raisins and orange

Red cabbage is an undervalued vegetable but its bright rich color works well and looks great with most meats but particularly game and poultry. It would work well with Stuffed Quail (page 99) or Mediterranean Chicken (page 104). **Serves 6**

1¾ lbs. red cabbage
3 tablespoons olive oil
2 tablespoons dark soft brown sugar
2 medium apples, peeled, cored and cubed

Grated zest and juice of 1 large orange
1¼ cups raisins or golden raisins
Salt and freshly ground black pepper
⅓ cup balsamic vinegar

Cut the cabbage in half, cut out the hard, thick white core and discard, then finely slice. Heat the olive oil in a large saucepan and gently braise the cabbage on a medium heat for 5 minutes, stirring occasionally. You do not want to brown the cabbage—just glaze it with oil. Add ⅔ cup water, the sugar, apples, orange zest and juice, raisins or golden raisins, and season with salt and pepper. Place a lid on the saucepan and cook gently for about 45 minutes, stirring the cabbage periodically and checking that there is enough liquid to prevent it "catching" the base of the pan. After the cabbage is just tender, remove the lid from the pan and add the balsamic vinegar. Carry on cooking for another 10 minutes until all the liquid has evaporated and the cabbage has a nice sugary glaze. **Serve** immediately or allow to cool and store for up to 4 days in the fridge for reheating as required.

Fiber rating: HIGH
Per serving: 5.2g fiber, 215 Calories, 6g fat, 1g saturated fat, 0.33g sodium

Spinach with sesame sauce Japanese style

A simple but interesting way of serving spinach. It goes well with steamed fish or with other Japanese-style recipes in this book, such as Mackerel Simmered in Miso Soup (see page 88). **Serves 4**

9 cups (1³/₄ lbs.) spinach	1 tablespoon soy sauce
1 teaspoon finely grated fresh ginger root	1 tablespoon water or 2 tablespoons chicken stock
1 large garlic clove, finely grated	2 tablespoons black or yellow sesame seeds
1 tablespoon tahini (sesame paste)	

Wash the spinach and trim off any large thick stems, but don't bother if they are thin and not too long. Cook the spinach in a large saucepan, stirring frequently—you will probably not need any more water than is clinging to the leaves. Rinse in cold water to cool and squeeze well so the spinach is not soggy.

Place the ginger and garlic in the bottom of a bowl big enough to hold the spinach as well. Stir the tahini first (as it often separates when left to stand) and add to the bowl along with the soy sauce and water or chicken stock. Mix well and add the spinach.

Mix all the ingredients together, taste for the correct balance of seasoning and serve mounded high on a plate with a scattering of sesame seeds on top.

Fiber rating: HIGH
Per serving: 5.5g fiber, 147 Calories, 11g fat, 1g saturated fat, 0.45g sodium

Roasted winter vegetables with barley

A variety of vegetables can be used for this recipe, including sweet potatoes, celery root, pumpkin, and turnips. It is quite high in fat due to the olive oil used, so is best avoided if you are following a low-fat diet. **Serves 4**

³/₄ cup barley	3 medium red onions
5 garlic cloves	4 medium leeks
4 heaping tablespoons chopped sage or thyme, plus 1 small sprig	7 tablespoons extra virgin olive oil
Salt and freshly ground pepper	1 tablespoon lemon juice
14oz. pumpkin	¹/₃ cup almonds, toasted in a medium oven for 10 minutes until brown
3–4 medium zucchini	

Rinse the barley, place in a saucepan and cover with water. Bring to a boil, drain and rinse again. Place back in the saucepan with 1 of the garlic cloves, the herb sprig, and fresh water to cover. Bring to a boil and simmer gently for 45 minutes to 1 hour, making sure there is always enough water to cover the barley. The barley should be just soft. Season with salt, drain and set aside. Reheat if need be just before serving.

Preheat the oven to 400°F. Peel the pumpkin and cut it and the zucchini into large wedges. Cut the onions in half or quarters, depending on their size, and the leeks in half. Mix all the vegetables with the remaining 4 garlic cloves (unpeeled), 3 tablespoons of the olive oil, salt and pepper. Place the vegetables in a roasting pan and roast for about 45 minutes until soft, checking them halfway through the cooking time.

Make a sauce with the chopped sage or thyme, a good pinch of salt, pepper, the lemon juice, and the remaining olive oil in a food processor. Set aside.

When the barley and vegetables are cooked, spoon 1 tablespoon of the sage sauce into the barley and season if need be.

Place a spoonful of the barley on each serving plate and arrange a variety of the vegetables on top. Finally drizzle over the rest of the sauce, scatter with almonds and serve.

Fiber rating: HIGH
Per serving: 6.9g fiber, 344 Calories, 29g fat, 4g saturated fat, 0.3g sodium

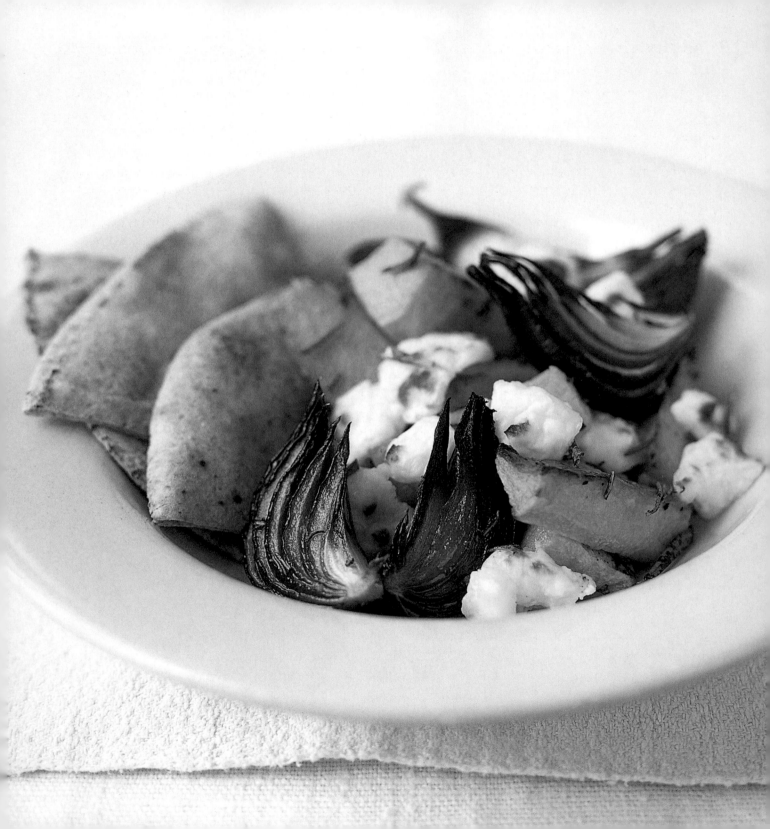

Roast butternut squash and onions with feta

A lovely vegetarian dish, ideal for a light lunch, evening meal or appetizer. It can be prepared in advance and assembled just before serving. Other kinds of pumpkin can be used in this recipe. **Serves 6**

2¼ lbs. butternut squash, peeled and seeded

3 large red onions

8 garlic cloves

1 small bunch sage or rosemary, coarsely chopped

Salt and freshly ground black pepper

5 tablespoons extra virgin olive oil

1⅓ cups feta cheese

To serve

4 wholewheat pita or Lebanese flatbread, toasted, and salad

Preheat the oven to 350°F.

Cut the squash and onions into wedges and place separately on aluminum foil-lined baking sheets. Scatter over the garlic and sage or rosemary and season with salt and pepper. Drizzle 4 tablespoons of the oil over the vegetables and bake them in the oven for about 30 minutes or until the squash is soft. The onions might take a little longer to cook, so just remove the pumpkin and carry on cooking the onions. Once both vegetables are cooked, set aside. This can be done in advance and the vegetables reheated later.

Preheat the grill to high. Place the vegetables in a gratin dish or on a heat-proof plate. Break the feta into small cubes and sprinkle over the vegetables. Drizzle the remaining tablespoon of olive oil over the feta and broil until the cheese is light golden brown.

Serve with toasted pita or flatbread and a little salad.

Fiber rating: HIGH
Per serving including wholewheat pita bread: 6.8g fiber, 400 Calories, 17g fat, 6g saturated fat, 0.72g sodium

Roasted celery root, tomatoes, and olives

A high-fiber vegetable dish to serve with simply broiled or roasted meat to bring fiber into the meal. Great in the fall or winter when celery root is in season. Its mild, sweet flavor contrasts well with the olives and rosemary. **Serves 4**

1¼ lbs. celery root

5 medium ripe tomatoes

16 pitted black olives, halved

1 heaping tablespoon chopped rosemary

2 large garlic cloves, chopped

4 tablespoons extra virgin olive oil

Salt and freshly ground black pepper

Preheat the oven to 400°F.

Trim the celery root, removing the skin, and cut into 1-inch cubes. Cut the tomatoes into large chunks and place in a bowl with the celery root, olives, rosemary, garlic, olive oil, salt and pepper. Mix well.

Place the vegetables in a gratin dish about 10 x 15 inches, so that they are not overcrowded. Bake in the oven for about 45 minutes to 1 hour, until the vegetables are golden brown and soft.

Serve with simply broiled meat.

Fiber rating: HIGH
Per serving: 6.2g fiber, 149 Calories, 13g fat, 2g saturated fat, 0.73g sodium

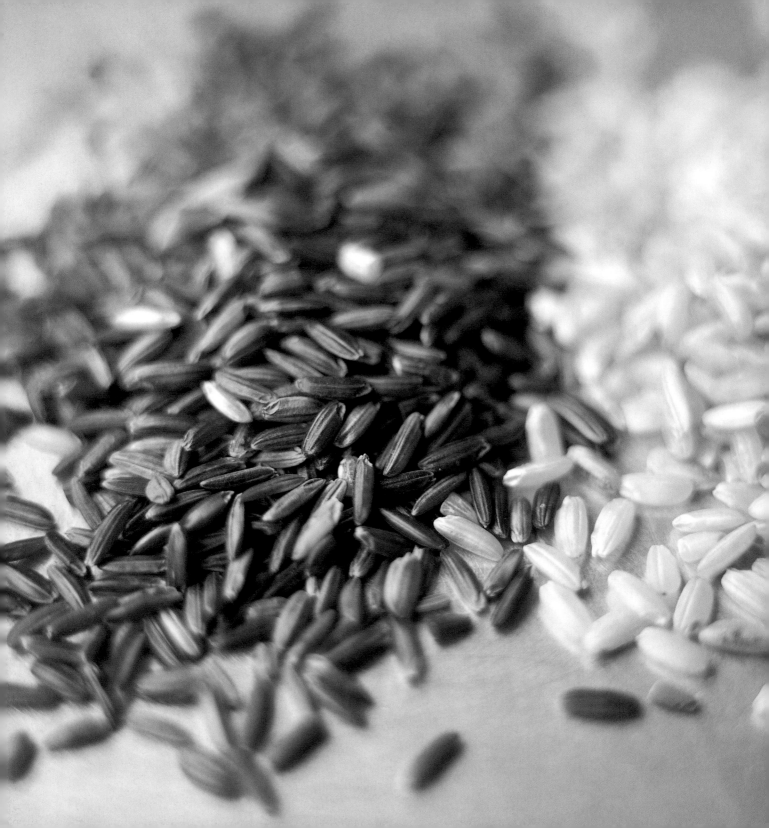

7 Pasta, Rice, and Pulses

Pumpkin risotto
This is a really comforting dish which is best in fall when pumpkins are in season. Use a sweet, flavorful pumpkin such as butternut squash or a Turkish turban. Avoid the pumpkins produced for decoration, which can be watery and tasteless. **Serves 4**

6 tablespoons extra virgin olive oil

1 medium onion, finely chopped

19oz. pumpkin, peeled and cut into small cubes

1 large clove garlic, chopped

3 cups chicken stock, preferably homemade

Pinch of grated nutmeg

2 tablespoons chopped sage

1¼ cups risotto rice, e.g., arborio or carnaroli

Salt and freshly ground black pepper

⅓ cup dry white vermouth or white wine

5 tablespoons grated Parmesan cheese,

Heat the oil in a heavy saucepan and gently cook the onion, pumpkin, and garlic for about 20 minutes until soft, without coloring. Heat the chicken stock in another saucepan.

Add the nutmeg, sage, and rice to the pumpkin and mix briefly. Season with salt and pepper and stir for 1 minute to coat the grains of rice.

Add the vermouth or wine and increase the heat to medium. Keep stirring the rice, and when the liquid has almost absorbed into the rice, start adding the hot stock, a couple of ladles at a time, stirring the rice all the time so that it cooks evenly and releases some of its starch, making a creamy consistency.

Taste the liquid around the rice for enough seasoning after adding the first couple of ladles of stock, while the rice is still absorbing flavor. Add more salt and pepper if need be.

When you have nearly used up the stock, start tasting the rice to prevent overcooking. It is ready when it is "al dente." Add more water or stock as necessary but stop cooking the rice as soon as it still has a little texture in the middle of the grain. The consistency of the risotto should be rich and thick like porridge, not too sloppy or too dry. Add half the Parmesan just before serving and hand round the rest separately for sprinkling.

Fiber rating: LOW
Per serving: 1.5g fiber, 403 Calories, 20g fat, 4g saturated fat, 0.89g sodium

Pasta with clams
An attractive informal dinner party dish as the pretty shells are left in. In Italy it wouldn't be the done thing to serve this with cheese as it contains chile and fish. There is no need to add any extra salt to this dish (apart from to the pasta water) as the clams are salty enough. **Serves 4**

2¼ lbs. clams, cleaned and drained

Salt

⅓ cup white wine

3 cups spaghetti or linguine

4 tablespoons extra virgin olive oil

2 large garlic cloves, finely chopped

1 large red chile, finely chopped

3 heaping tablespoons coarsely chopped cilantro

Rinse the clams in cold water. Leave in the water for a few minutes, then drain well.

Bring a large saucepan of salted water to a boil. Heat a large sauté pan or skillet with a lid for the clams.

With all the ingredients on hand, add the clams to the hot sauté pan, pour in the wine and cover with a lid. Cook for about 1 minute until all the clams have opened, then drain in a colander placed over a bowl to collect the juice. (You can cook in batches if your pan is not big enought to cook them all at once.)

Add the pasta to the salted boiling water, stirring well to prevent the strands of pasta sticking together. Cook according to the packet instructions until al dente.

Heat the oil in the empty sauté pan and cook the garlic and chile briefly, then add the cilantro and the clam juice, reserving and discarding any sediment. Cook briefly to concentrate the flavors.

Drain the pasta well, add to the sauté pan off the heat and mix thoroughly. Add the clams at the last minute.

Serve immediately, dividing up the pasta and then the clams for easiest results. Pour any remaining juice over each portion.

Fiber rating: LOW
Per serving: 2.3g fiber, 419 Calories, 13g fat, 2g saturated fat, 1.25g sodium

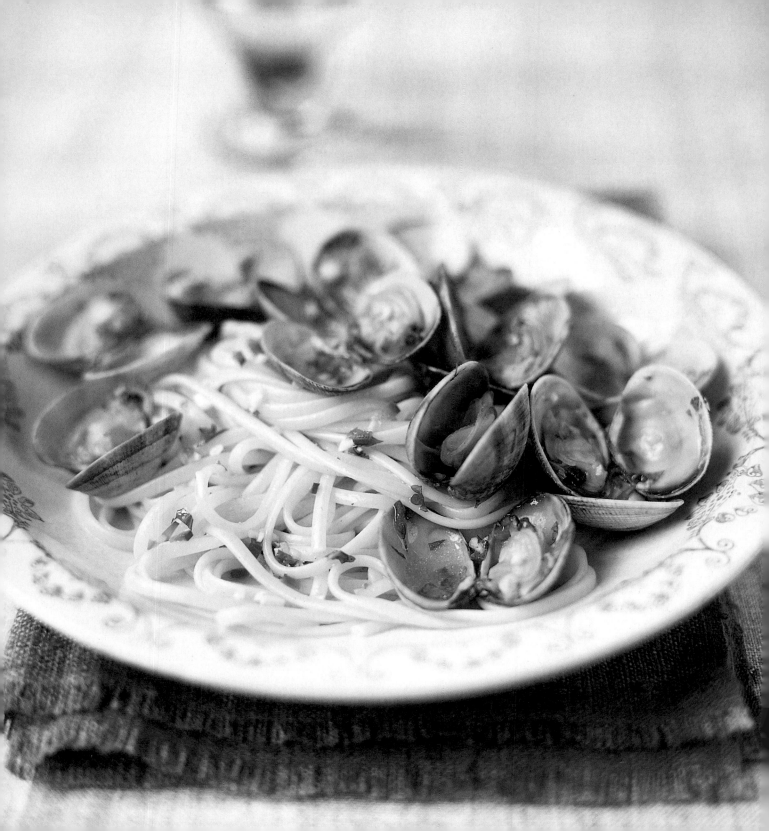

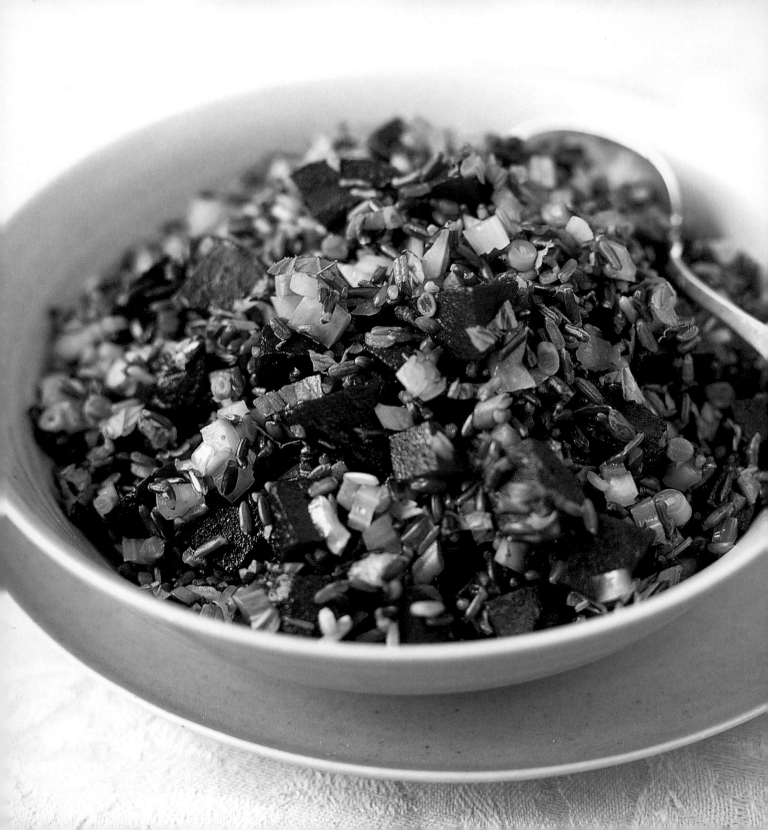

Red rice with green beans and beets

This dish can be served hot or at room temperature as a salad. With its vibrant colors this complements any grilled meat or fish or alternatively can be served as a vegetarian main course. Serves 4

1 cup red rice
2 garlic cloves (unpeeled)
Salt and freshly ground black pepper
2 tablespoons extra virgin olive oil
1 medium onion, finely chopped
2 celery sticks, finely chopped

½ cup green beans, topped, tailed and cut into discs
Pinch of ground allspice (optional)
7oz. cooked beets (not in vinegar), cut into ½-inch cubes
2 heaping tablespoons coarsely chopped mint

Rinse the rice and then cook in a generous amount of boiling water with the garlic and a pinch of salt for about 40 minutes until soft but with a little nutty bite to it still. Drain well.

Heat the oil and cook the onion, celery, and green beans for about 10 minutes until they are soft. Add the rice and allspice, if using, and mix well. Season with salt and pepper. Add the beets and mint at the last minute, mix briefly and serve hot or leave to cool at room temperature.

Fiber rating: MEDIUM
Per serving: 3.4g fiber, 270 Calories, 7g fat, 1g saturated fat, 0.57g sodium

Borlotti bean salad with broccoli, pine nuts, and anchovies

This can be a meal in itself or can accompany fish or meat. Serve with warm crusty wholewheat bread for extra fiber. **Serves 2 as a main dish or 4 as a side dish**

2½ cups broccoli
¼ cup pine nuts, roasted for 10 minutes in medium oven
1oz. canned anchovies, drained and chopped
14-oz. can borlotti beans, drained and rinsed
2 heaping tablespoons chopped mixed fresh herbs such as parsley, mint, and basil

Juice of ½ lemon
3 tablespoons extra virgin olive oil
Salt and freshly ground black pepper
Wholewheat bread for serving (optional)

Steam or boil the broccoli until just tender. Drain well and place in a large bowl with the pine nuts, anchovies, and borlotti beans.

Just before serving add the herbs, lemon juice, olive oil, and season with salt and pepper. Mix well and serve.

Fiber rating: MEDIUM
Per serving (side dish) not including bread: 3.9g fiber, 203 Calories, 14g fat, 2g saturated fat, 0.68g sodium

Saffron and raisin rice

A Middle Eastern recipe where rice is combined with lots of other ingredients, but particularly dried fruits, to give it a sort of sweet and sour flavor. Delicious served with Garam Masala Duck (see page 98). Serves 4–6

1¼ cups brown basmati rice

4 tablespoons extra virgin olive oil

1 medium onion, finely chopped

3½ oz. shelled pistachio nuts or pine nuts

2 teaspoons cumin seeds

½ cup raisins

6 whole cardamom pods

1 small cinnamon stick

Large pinch of saffron strands, soaked in a little water

Salt and freshly ground black pepper

Rinse the rice in a bowl of cold water and drain.

Pour the oil into a large saucepan or skillet, add the onion, nuts, and cumin seeds and cook on a medium heat until the onion is soft and the nuts and cumin have infused in the oil. Add the raisins, cardamom, cinnamon stick, rice, and saffron and season with salt and pepper. Briefly mix all the ingredients together and add enough water to cover the rice by about ¾-inch. Cook at a gentle simmer, covered with a lid, for about 30 minutes.

Remove the pan from the heat and with the lid still sealed tight, leave to steam for another 5 minutes until the rice is cooked and the liquid has evaporated. If need be, remove the lid and gently cook the rice until no liquid remains.

Serve hot or at room temperature.

Fiber rating: MEDIUM
Per serving (4 people): 3.6g fiber, 637 Calories, 27g fat, 4g saturated fat, 0.34g sodium

Thai-style squid and chickpea salad

Pulses are not traditionally used in Thai cooking, but chickpeas work very well with squid and I've always loved how the Thais make refreshing squid salads. So I've fused two great recipes to create a tasty medium-fiber salad. Serves 4

2 medium squid, 1¾ lbs. total weight

2 tablespoons sunflower oil

3½ oz. scallions or red onions, thinly sliced

2 heaping teaspoons finely chopped fresh ginger root

2 garlic cloves, finely chopped

½ large red chile, finely chopped (optional)

8½ oz. cooked chickpeas or 14-oz. can, rinsed and drained

Juice of 1 lime (3 tablespoons)

1 tablespoon Thai fish sauce

2 heaping tablespoons coarsely chopped cilantro

1 large tomato, cubed

Get your fish merchant to gut and clean the squid, removing the skin and wings as well. Cut through the body of the squid to flatten out and wash well, making sure the tentacles have all the grit and sand removed from the suckers. Cut into thin strips and drain well.

Prepare all the ingredients before cooking. Heat the oil in a large wok or sauté pan until hot. Add the drained squid and cook, stirring frequently, for about 1–2 minutes, depending on the thickness. Push to one side and add the onions, ginger, garlic, and chile, if using. Turn the heat down to medium and cook for 1 minute. Add the chickpeas, stirring well, and cook 1 further minute.

Remove the pan from the heat and add the lime juice, fish sauce, and cilantro. Mix well and transfer to a serving bowl, add the tomato and serve hot or at room temperature.

Fiber rating: MEDIUM
Per serving: 3.3g fiber, 226 Calories, 9g fat, 1g saturated fat, 0.54g sodium

Buckwheat pasta with spinach, mushrooms, and truffle oil

Buckwheat pasta is often used in Italian cooking. Like faro, it's a good substitute for wheat pasta. If you are unable to find truffle oil, use a tablespoon of crème fraîche or creamy goat cheese instead. **Serves 4**

- 2 tablespoons extra virgin olive oil
- 4½ oz. chestnut or shiitake mushrooms
- 1 large garlic clove, chopped
- 1 tablespoon chopped thyme or sage
- 2–3 cups (7oz.) small leaf spinach
- 3 cups buckwheat or faro (spelt) pasta
- Salt and freshly ground black pepper
- 2 heaping tablespoons grated Parmesan cheese
- Truffle oil, to serve (optional)

Heat the olive oil in a sauté pan or skillet and cook the mushrooms until soft. Add the garlic and thyme or sage and cook briefly, then add the spinach in batches, stirring the leaves well until they start to wilt before adding the next batch. Continue until the spinach is just cooked. Add a few tablespoons of water if the spinach becomes too dry. Set aside.

Bring a saucepan of salted water to a boil and cook the pasta according to the packet instructions until "al dente." Reserve a small cup of the cooking water and drain the pasta, then add the pasta to the spinach mixture. Mix well, adding a little of the reserved cooking water to stop the pasta from sticking and season with salt and pepper.

Serve right away sprinkled with Parmesan and a good drizzle of truffle oil.

Fiber rating: MEDIUM
Per serving: 4.7g fiber, 366 Calories, 9g fat, 2g saturated fat, 0.36g sodium

Chickpea stew with eggplant, zucchini, and tomatoes

This chickpea stew is even better eaten the next day as the flavors will intensify beautifully. Barley couscous is a good alternative to wheat couscous. Serves 4

- 12oz. eggplant, cut into 2-inch cubes
- 1 heaping tablespoon coriander seeds
- 1 heaping tablespoon cumin seeds
- 6 tablespoons extra virgin olive oil
- 1 medium onion, quartered and sliced
- 3 medium zucchini, cut into 1¼-inch cubes
- 1 large garlic clove
- Salt and freshly ground black pepper
- 14-oz. can chickpeas, rinsed and drained
- 3 smallish tomatoes, skinned and chopped

To serve (optional)
- 2 heaping tablespoons coarsely chopped fresh cilantro, couscous and low-fat live yogurt

Salt the eggplant cubes generously, and leave in a bowl to "sweat" for 15 minutes. Rinse in cold water to remove the salt and any bitter juices and squeeze dry.

Gently dry-roast the coriander and cumin seeds in a heavy skillet until they give off an aroma. Grind using a mortar and pestle or spice grinder.

Heat the olive oil into a large skillet or sauté pan and cook the eggplant on a medium-high heat on all sides, until golden brown and soft. Remove from the pan and set aside to drain.

Cook the onion, zucchini, and garlic in the same pan for about 15 minutes until the onion is soft and the zucchini are light golden brown. Season with salt and pepper and add the chickpeas and ground spices. Mix briefly and add the tomatoes. Cover and simmer for a further 15 minutes, until the flavors have amalgamated and the tomatoes reduced a little.

Allow to infuse for at least 15 minutes for a better flavor before serving with chopped fresh cilantro, couscous, and yogurt.

Fiber rating: HIGH
Per serving not including serving suggestion: 6.2g fiber, 270 Calories, 20g fat, 3g saturated fat, 0.43g sodium

Wild rice and spelt with chestnuts and sesame seeds

A tasty side dish that experiments with unusual starches. Wild rice is in fact a grass as opposed to a "proper" rice. Buy packets or cans of peeled and cooked chestnuts to make this dish easy to prepare. **Serves 6**

1¼ cups wild rice

5oz. spelt or faro

2 large garlic cloves

2 tablespoons sesame or sunflower oil

1 medium onion, chopped

2 heaping tablespoons sesame seeds

7oz. cooked peeled chestnuts, coarsely chopped

Boil the rice and spelt together with a pinch of salt and the whole garlic cloves in plenty of water for 45 minutes, until the rice and spelt are cooked but still have a bit of bite. Drain well and remove the skin from the garlic.

Heat the oil in a saucepan and gently cook the onion for 5 minutes. Add the sesame seeds, mix well and cook for a further 5 minutes, until the onion is soft and the sesame seeds light golden brown. Stir frequently.

Add the chopped chestnuts and mix briefly. Then add the rice and warm through, mixing all the flavors together and breaking up the soft garlic.

Serve hot or at room temperature.

Fiber rating: HIGH

Per serving: 5.2g fiber, 377 Calories, 9g fat, 1g saturated fat, 0g sodium

Faro pasta salad with tomatoes, cannellini beans, and basil

Faro pasta is made from spelt, a grain often used in Italian cooking. For best results, use shaped pasta rather than strands. They are less gluey so work better in cold pasta salads. **Serves 6**

2½ cups fusilli faro pasta

Salt and freshly ground black pepper

4½ oz. cooked cannellini beans, rinsed and drained

3 medium tasty tomatoes, cubed

4 tablespoons chopped or torn basil

1 large garlic clove, crushed with salt

3 scallions, finely chopped

2 tablespoons sherry vinegar

4 tablespoons extra virgin olive oil

Cook the pasta in a large saucepan of salted boiling water until al dente. Allow about 7 minutes or follow the packet instructions. Drain, refresh under cold water and drain well again.

Place the cannellini beans in a bowl. Add the cubed tomatoes, basil, and garlic crushed with salt. Add the scallions, vinegar, and oil and season with pepper and a little more salt if need be. Mix in the pasta, taste for seasoning and leave to infuse for a few minutes before serving.

Fiber rating: HIGH

Per serving: 6.1g fiber, 280 Calories, 9g fat, 1g saturated fat, 0.33g sodium

Lentil salad with bacon and broiled peppers

This is what I call an all-in-one salad because it includes carbohydrates in the form of lentils. Green or Puy lentils are a good alternative to serving rice or potatoes with any dish. They are easy to cook, and can be prepared in advance. **Serves 4**

1 tablespoon extra virgin
  olive oil
1 cup smoked bacon or
  pancetta, cubed
2 medium carrots, finely
  chopped
1 large celery stalk, finely
  chopped
1 large garlic clove, finely
  chopped
1 tablespoon chopped
  rosemary
1½ cups Puy or green lentils

To serve
1–1½ cups small leaf spinach
7oz. endive lettuce, cut
  in half
3 tablespoons lemon juice
1 tablespoon extra virgin
  olive oil
Salt and freshly ground black
  pepper
2 red bell peppers, broiled,
  seeded and cut into strips
  (optional)

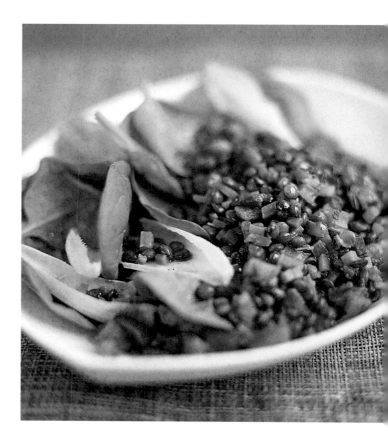

Heat the oil in a saucepan and cook the bacon or pancetta until golden and crispy. Add the carrots, celery, garlic, and rosemary and cook gently for about 10 minutes.

Add the lentils, mix briefly, then add 2 cups water. Cover with a lid and simmer gently for about 1–1½ hours until the lentils are cooked and all the water has evaporated.

When you are ready to serve, place the salad leaves on individual serving plates or one large plate. Drizzle over the lemon juice and oil, season with salt and pepper and mix briefly. Scatter over the lentils and top with the strips of red peppers, if using. Serve right away.

Fiber rating: HIGH
Per serving, including peppers: 7.2g fiber, 288 Calories, 13g fat,
3g saturated fat, 0.7g sodium

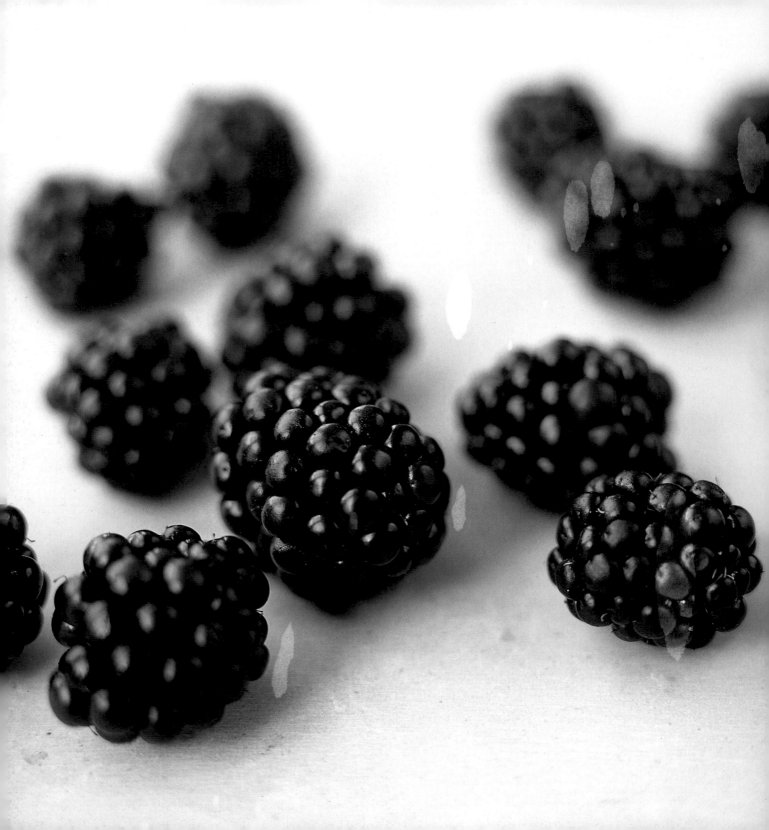

8

Desserts

Peach and grappa sorbet

The best results are achieved when good tasty peaches are in season. Other summer fruits can be substituted and a different alcohol used. Increase the sugar quantity if the mixture is too acidic or add more fruit purée or lemon juice if it is too sweet. **Serves 6**

5 heaping tablespoons superfine sugar

5 tablespoons grappa or brandy (or water if preferred)

5 large peaches, skinned, pitted and chopped

Juice of 1 large lemon

Place the sugar and alcohol or water in a small saucepan and heat gently until the sugar has dissolved. Set aside.

Put the peaches and lemon juice in a food processor and purée finely. Do not over-purée or the color of the peaches will deteriorate, though the lemon juice helps to prevent this. Pour the peach purée—there should be about 4 cups—into a bowl, add the sugar and alcohol syrup and mix thoroughly.

Place in an ice-cream maker and freeze according to the manufacturer's instructions.

If you don't have an ice-cream maker, place the sorbet in a metal bowl or plastic container and place in the freezer. Remove every 30 minutes, stirring well to churn the sorbet into a creamy consistency. Continue this process until it is set. **If** not eating right away, freeze the sorbet immediately as peach juice will oxidize, turning an unattractive brown color.

Fiber rating: LOW
Per serving: 1.9g fiber, 124 Calories, 0g fat, 0g saturated fat, 0g sodium

Strawberry cheesecake

Quark is a fresh curd cheese made from skim milk and, as it has a neutral taste, it is ideal for use in desserts like this one. Quark is used here to keep the fat content down, but you can substitute cream cheese if you feel like being indulgent. **Serves 6**

7oz. Graham crackers

2/3 cup blanched almonds, roasted in a medium oven for 10 minutes

6 tablespoons butter, melted

18oz. quark

2 heaping tablespoons confectioners' sugar, or to taste

Grated zest of 1 orange

1 cup hulled strawberries

1 heaping tablespoon superfine or confectioners' sugar

1 tablespoon orange juice

Roughly break up the Graham crackers and grind in a food processor with half the almonds. Mix in the melted butter. Line an 8-inch springform pan (non-fluted) with plastic wrap. Put the cracker mixture into the pan and press down firmly into the base and push up a little around the sides. Place in the fridge to set for 1 hour.

Place the quark in a bowl. Coarsely chop the remaining almonds and add to the quark along with the confectioners' sugar and orange zest. Taste for sweetness. Place on top of the cracker base, spreading to cover all edges. Leave to rest in the fridge for another hour before serving.

To make the topping, cut the strawberries in quarters or smaller pieces, depending on their size. Mix with the sugar and orange juice and leave to marinate.

Remove the cheesecake from the pan, carefully peeling off the plastic wrap before placing it on a plate. Pour the strawberries over the top of the cheesecake just before serving.

Fiber rating: LOW
Per serving: 2.4g fiber, 449 Calories, 26g fat, 10g saturated fat, 0.31g sodium

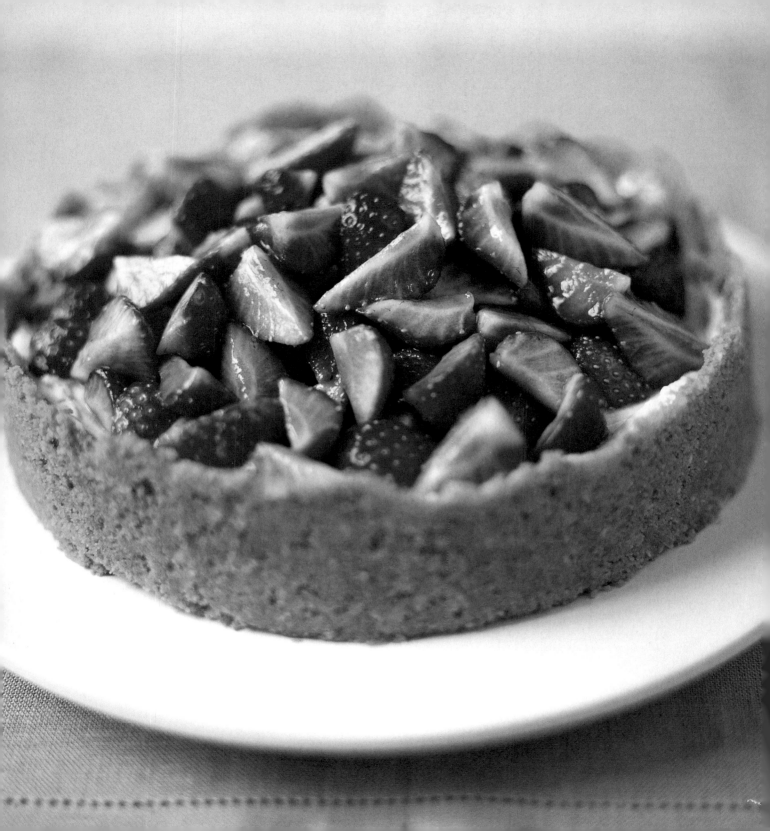

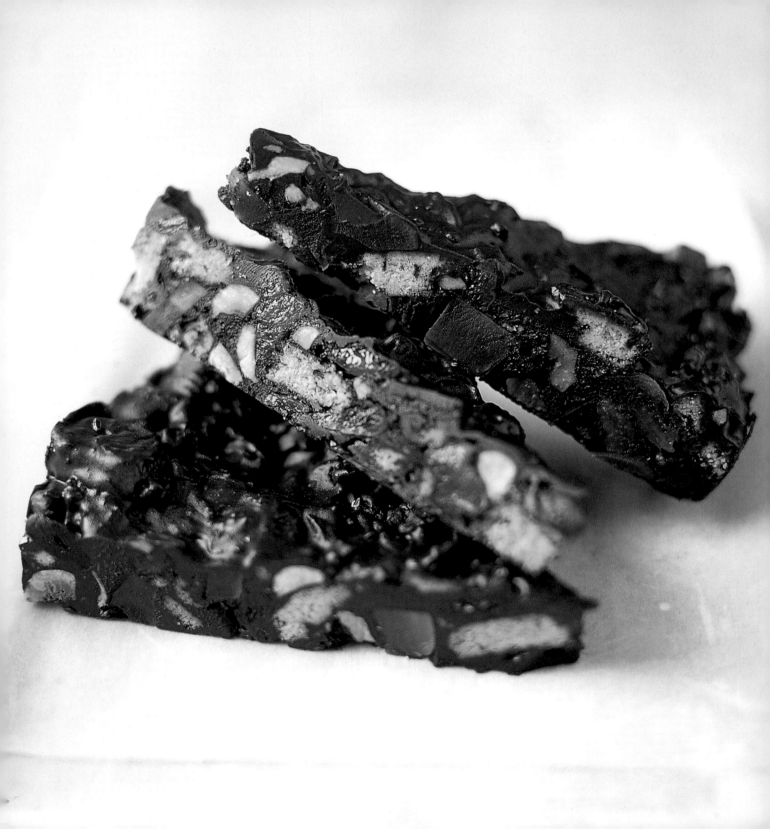

Chocolate fridge cake

This is my sophisticated version of the timeless cake. Any dried fruit can be used such as pineapple, pears, or apples. If you prefer your desserts sweeter, add 1oz. unrefined sugar when melting the chocolate and butter. But don't buy cheap sweet chocolate! **Serves 6–8**

½ cup hazelnuts
5oz. dried fruit, such as cranberries, apricots, and papaya
5 tablespoons brandy or rum

6oz. plain chocolate, 70% cocoa solids, cut into small pieces
6 tablespoons unsalted butter, cubed
3oz. Graham crackers

Line an 8-inch cake pan generously with plastic wrap, so that it reaches over the sides.

Roast the nuts in a medium-high oven for 10 minutes until golden brown. Chop coarsely and place in a large bowl.

Cut the fruit, if need be, into small pieces and mix with the brandy or rum. Set aside to marinate.

Melt the chocolate and butter in a bowl set over a pan of gently simmering water, making sure the base of the bowl does not touch the water, or in a microwave on medium-high. Mix briefly, being careful not to over-heat the chocolate or it will become grainy, not smooth.

Break the Graham crackers into small pieces and add to the nuts. Pour over the chocolate mixture and add the dried fruits. Mix well.

Pour the chocolate mixture into the pan, pressing down to keep it compact. Cover the pan with plastic wrap, making sure it does not touch the top of the mixture, and place in the fridge for at least 4 hours or overnight until chilled and solid. Serve cool.

Fiber rating: MEDIUM
Per serving (6 people): 3g fiber, 430 Calories, 26g fat, 13g saturated fat, 0.09g sodium

Almond and polenta cookies with fresh fruit

These easy cookies are a great way to make a plate of fresh fruit more interesting. I use whole almonds when cooking, because ground almonds tend to go stale more quickly. **Makes 24 small cookies**

⅔ cup blanched almonds
1 heaping cup wholewheat flour
½ cup superfine sugar
⅔ cup cornmeal or polenta
Grated zest of 1 orange
2 medium eggs

⅓ cup sunflower oil
1 level teaspoon baking powder
To serve
Confectioners' sugar, to decorate (optional)
½ passionfruit and 3-oz. slice pineapple per person

Preheat the oven to 350°F.

Place all the ingredients, except the confectioners' sugar and fruit, in a food processor and blend until the nuts are finely ground.

Line two baking sheets with baking parchment. Space half tablespoons of the mixture evenly on the prepared sheets, forming each into a slightly oval shape, ensuring that there is a slight gap between each to allow them to spread while cooking.

Bake in the oven for 15–20 minutes. Remove from the oven and leave to rest on the sheet for a further 10 minutes until cool enough to handle.

Dust the cookies with a little confectioners' sugar if you wish and serve at room temperature with fresh seasonal fruit.

Fiber rating: MEDIUM
Per 2 cookies with fruit: 3.1g fiber, 277 Calories, 15g fat, 2g saturated fat, 0.05g sodium

Caramelized pears with walnuts and raisins
A simple dessert which is lovely and warming with the addition of cinnamon and ginger. It can be served with yogurt and a high-fiber cookie such as a flapjack to increase the fiber content. **Serves 4**

4 large slightly ripe pears
½ stick unsalted butter
2 tablespoons unrefined superfine sugar
Pinch each of cinnamon and ground ginger

¾ cup walnut pieces
2oz. raisins or dried cranberries
2 tablespoons lemon juice
Low-fat live yogurt, to serve

Cut the pears in quarters and remove the core. In a large skillet or sauté pan, gently melt the butter and add the sugar. Place the pears on top and sprinkle with the cinnamon and ginger. Bring to a gentle simmer to cook the pears, carefully turning and moving them so all get a light browning. Cover with a lid to half-steam and prevent the sugar browning too quickly before the pears are cooked. Alternatively add a dash of water if using a skillet. Cook for about 20 minutes, until the fruit is soft.

Carefully remove the pears, one at a time, to a serving plate. Add the walnut pieces and raisins or cranberries to the pan and cook for 5 minutes, stirring to prevent the sugar from crystallizing. (Alternatively the walnuts can be toasted in a medium oven for 10 minutes and added to the pears at the end.) Add the lemon juice (this can be added earlier if the butter has been absorbed and the sugar is starting to caramelize).

Cover the pears with the nuts and dried fruit and serve while still warm with a dollop of yogurt.

Fiber rating: HIGH
Per serving including yogurt: 5.9g fiber, 386 Calories, 24g fat, 8g saturated fat, 0.04g sodium

Black currant fool
A simple dessert that uses labnah or strained yogurt to make a thicker fool than ordinary thick yogurt would make. The black currants are left whole to retain the fiber which is in their skins. If not using meringues, you might want to increase the quantity of sugar to 3oz. **Serves 4**

4 tablespoons unrefined sugar
4 tablespoons elderflower cordial or crème de cassis
14oz. black currants (the ready-made frozen ones are easiest to use)

9½ oz. labnah or strained yogurt (see page 74)
2 large meringue nests or 4 small meringues, or Almond and Polenta Cookies (see page 137), to serve

Dissolve the sugar in the elderflower cordial or crème de cassis in a saucepan over a gentle heat.

Mix the sugar liquid with the black currants and purée well in a food processor. Allow to cool, then add the labnah or strained yogurt. Mix briefly and taste to check for the right balance of sweetness and sharpness.

If using meringues, break up into bite-sized pieces and place in the bottom of four pretty glasses or ramekins or small bowls. Spoon over the black currant fool and serve right away or no more than 1 hour later—don't prepare too far in advance or the meringue will become too soft and gooey.

If serving with cookies, place the fool in glasses or bowls, cover with plastic wrap and leave in the fridge to firm up for several hours beforehand.

Fiber rating: MEDIUM
Per serving with meringue: 3.6g fiber, 145 Calories, 1g fat, 0g saturated fat, 0.05g sodium

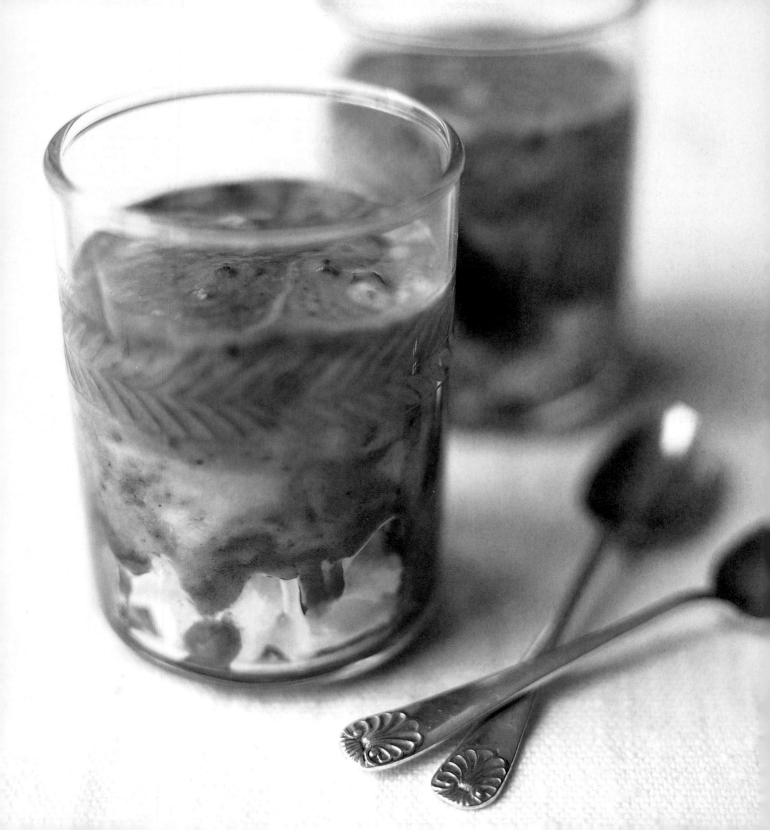

Date-filled sticky toffee pudding

This might not be the healthiest of desserts, but at least it is high in fiber! The darker the sugar, the darker-looking the sponge. I find that yogurt works very well with this pudding as it balances the sweetness of the sauce. **Serves 6**

1 cup pitted dates, finely chopped
1 stick plus 1 tablespoon unsalted butter, softened
¾ cup dark soft brown sugar
2 medium eggs
1 cup wholewheat flour
1 cup bran
1 teaspoon baking powder

For the sauce
½ cup dark soft brown sugar
6 tablespoons unsalted butter
3 tablespoons heavy cream
Low-fat live yogurt or heavy cream, to serve (optional)

First make the sauce by placing all the ingredients in a saucepan and melting slowly over a very low heat until the sugar has dissolved, then simmer gently for 1 minute. Pour the mixture into the base of a 18-oz. loaf pan or individual ramekins or dariole molds. Set aside to cool.

Preheat the oven to 350°F.

Place the dates in a saucepan with ¾ cup water and bring to a boil. Simmer for about 5 minutes until the dates have softened and the liquid completely evaporated. Set aside to cool.

Cream the butter and sugar until it becomes paler in color and then add the eggs one at a time, beating well. Add the flour, bran, baking powder, and cooled dates and gently fold in. Spoon this mixture on top of the sauce in the pan(s) and bake in the oven for about 20–40 minutes, depending on the size of the pan(s). Check every 10–15 minutes: when firm to the touch and a knife comes out clean when carefully placed into the center, the sponge is cooked.

Turn the pan(s) upside down to unmold the sponge and serve with either yogurt or cream, if you like.

Fiber rating: HIGH
Per serving not including yogurt or cream to serve: 5.4g fiber, 648 Calories, 42g fat, 26g saturated fat, 0.13g sodium

Wholewheat plum crumble

A simple crumble with added goodies to make it healthy. Substitute apricots for the plums if you wish; use fruit that is in season and that suits your fiber needs. For a lower fiber option you could use white flour instead of wholewheat flour. **Serves 4**

1 pound ripe plums
2 tablespoons unrefined superfine sugar (optional)
Low-fat live yogurt or vanilla ice cream, to serve (optional)

For the crumble topping
1 cup wholewheat flour
1 heaping tablespoon bran
½ cup rolled oats
2½ tablespoons sesame seeds
4 tablespoons unrefined superfine sugar
½ teaspoon ground cinnamon or ginger
2½ oz. sunflower margarine, cut into small pieces
5 tablespoons butter, cut into small pieces

Preheat the oven to 350°F.

Cut the plums in half and remove the pits. Place the plums in a 9 x 7 inches gratin dish and sprinkle over the sugar, if using.

To make the topping, place the dry ingredients in a bowl and, using the tips of your fingers, rub in the margarine and butter to create a coarse meal consistency. Scatter over the plums and bake in the oven for about 30 minutes, until the fruit is soft and the crumble golden brown.

Serve with a dollop of yogurt, or vanilla ice cream if you are allowed.

Fiber rating: HIGH
Per serving: 6.4g fiber, 475 Calories, 30g fat, 14g saturated fat, 0.18g sodium

Fig and cranberry bistaya cake

This "cake" is inspired by one from Morocco, where a pastry similar to phyllo is filled with savory as well as sweet fillings. The ingredients make it quite Christmassy, but it can be enjoyed at any time of year. Use fresh pears or apples instead of figs if you prefer. **Serves 6**

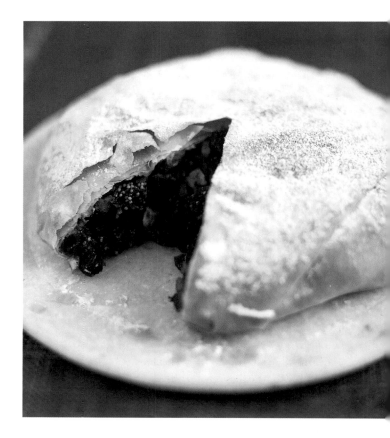

⅓ cup whole almonds or pistachio nuts

1 cup dried cranberries

2⅓ cups dried figs, diced

2 tablespoons brown sugar

1 teaspoon ground cinnamon

1 piece chopped stem ginger

1 tablespoon syrup from the stem ginger

2 tablespoons lemon, orange or apple juice

4½ oz. phyllo pastry (about 10 small sheets or 6 large sheets)

2 tablespoons sunflower oil

Confectioners' sugar, to decorate

Preheat the oven to 300°F. Roast the nuts for about 10 minutes, until golden brown, then chop coarsely. Turn the oven up to 350°F, ready to bake the pastry.

Place the nuts, cranberries, figs, sugar, cinnamon, ginger, and lemon, orange or apple juice in a bowl and mix well. Set aside to infuse for at least 10 minutes.

Line a baking sheet with baking parchment. Place 1 large or 2 slightly overlapping smaller sheets of phyllo pastry on the sheet and brush with sunflower oil. Cover with 3 or 6 more sheets of phyllo, brushing each layer with oil.

Place the fruit mixture in the middle, spreading it out to form a circle about 8-inch diameter and leaving a good margin of pastry around the outside. Fold up the pastry like a circular envelope. Brush with oil and place 2 sheets of phyllo on top, oiling each layer and trimming the pastry as necessary if using large sheets. Tuck a little of the phyllo underneath the "cake" to create a neat top. Finally brush with oil and bake in the oven for about 30 minutes, until the pastry is a light golden brown.

Leave to cool and dust with confectioners' sugar before serving.

Fiber rating: HIGH

Per serving: 5.7g fiber, 348 Calories, 16g fat, 3g saturated fat, 0.1g sodium

Index

Resources

US

International Foundation for Functional Gastrointestinal Disorders (IFFGD)
PO Box 170864
Milwaukee, WI 53217-8076
Tel: 414 964 1799
iffgd@iffgd.org
www.iffgd.org

IBS Self Help Group (IBSGroup)
1440 Whalley Avenue, #145
New Haven, CT 06515
ibs@ibsgroup.org
www.ibsgroup.org

IBS Association (IBSA)
Address as IBSGroup (see above)
ibsa@ibsassociation.org
www.ibsassociation.org

CANADA
IBS Self Help Group (IBSGroup)
P.O. Box 94074
Toronto, Ontario M4N 3R1
ibs@ibsgroup.org
www.ibsgroup.org

IBS Association (IBSA)
Address as IBSGroup (see above)
ibsa@ibsassociation.org
www.ibsassociation.org

The Canadian Society of Intestinal Research
855 West 12th Avenue
Vancouver, British Columbia
V5Z 1M9
Tel: 604 875 4875
Toll-Free (in Canada): 1 866 600 4875
www.badgut.com

UK
The IBS Research Appeal
PO Box 18
Crowborough
East Sussex TN6 1ZY
www.ibsresearchupdate.org.uk
www.please-help-my-ibs.org

IBS Network
Northern General Hospital
Sheffield S5 7AU
info@ibsnetwork.org.uk
www.ibsnetwork.org.uk

Core
3 St Andrew's Place
London NW1 4LB
info@corecharity.org.uk
www.corecharity.org.uk

AUSTRALIA
IBIS Australia
PO Box 7092
Sippy Downs
Qld 7092
Tel: 1300 651 131
contact@ibis-australia.org
www.ibis-australia.org

Text copyright © 2005 Sophie Braimbridge and Erica Jankovich
Photography copyright © 2005 Tara Fisher
Book design copyright © 2005 Kyle Cathie Limited

Published in 2006 by
Stewart, Tabori & Chang
115 West 18th Street
New York, NY 10011
www.abramsbooks.com

First published in Great Britain in 2005 by Kyle Cathie Limited

Library of Congress Cataloging-in-Publication Data is on file with the Library of Congress.

ISBN: 1-58479-494-1

Printed in Singapore

10 9 8 7 6 5 4 3 2 1

First Printing

LA MARTINIÈRE
GROUPE